Quantitative Evaluation *of the* Impact *of the* Healthy Communities Initiative *in* Cincinnati

Soeren Mattke, Hangsheng Liu, Samuel Hirshman,
Saw H. Wah, Sydne Newberry

SPONSORED BY THE GENERAL ELECTRIC COMPANY

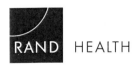

RAND HEALTH

For more information on this publication, visit www.rand.org/t/rr729

Library of Congress Cataloging-in-Publication Data is available for this publication.

ISBN: 978-0-8330-8754-6

Published by the RAND Corporation, Santa Monica, Calif.

© Copyright 2014 RAND Corporation

RAND® is a registered trademark.

Support RAND

Make a tax-deductible charitable contribution at
www.rand.org/giving/contribute

www.rand.org

Preface

Metropolitan Cincinnati residents have traditionally had among the highest health care costs in the United States, yet little evidence exists that residents are getting their money's worth, especially in terms of preventive and primary care. Recently, large employers, health plans, and health care providers in the Cincinnati area joined with community organizations in an effort to improve health care and population health, as well as reduce health care costs by focusing on five priority areas: coordinated primary care, health information exchange, quality improvement, public reporting and consumer engagement, and payment innovations. Spearheaded by General Electric (GE) Cincinnati, the resulting Healthy Communities Initiative in Cincinnati was implemented in 2009. In 2012, GE asked RAND Health Advisory Services to assess progress over the first three years of the initiative.

This research was conducted by RAND Health Advisory Services under Contract No. 2013-0573 to the GE Corporation. A profile of RAND Health, abstracts of its publications, and ordering information can be found at www.rand.org/health. Comments or inquiries concerning this report should be sent to the lead author, Soeren Mattke, at Soeren_Mattke@rand.org or to his address at RAND: RAND Corporation, 20 Park Plaza, Suite 920, Boston, MA 02116, phone +1 (617) 338 2059 x8622.

Table of Contents

Table of Contents

Table of Contents

Figures

Figures

Figures

Tables

Tables

Executive Summary

Background

Metropolitan Cincinnati residents have traditionally had among the highest health care costs in the United States, yet little evidence exists that people are getting their money's worth, especially in terms of preventive and primary care. On measures of misuse of care—such as emergency department (ED) visits or hospital admissions for conditions that should be managed in primary care settings, such as asthma—Cincinnati's rates are higher than rates in the state of Ohio or nationwide. Cincinnati also has higher rates of preventable mortality (Radley and Commonwealth Fund, 2012).

Recognizing that high health care spending was not resulting in a healthy population, community leaders began to prioritize local health care reform long before it became a national priority. Recently, large employers, health plans, and health care providers in the Cincinnati area joined with community organizations in a renewed effort to simultaneously lower costs and increase quality. Several factors unique to Cincinnati have spurred this initiative:

- the presence of several large employers (including General Electric [GE], Procter and Gamble, and The Kroger Co.) desiring to keep their employees healthy while controlling their health care costs
- changes to the health care infrastructure, including the consolidation of some hospitals and health care systems, resulting in a reduction in the number of players
- a long history of actively convening organizations comprising the business and health care communities (exemplified by the Health Collaborative, the Greater Cincinnati Health Council, and HealthBridge, which combined in 2012).

In 2009, GE's Healthy Communities Initiative in Cincinnati built on and revitalized this successful collaboration among employers, health plans, providers, and community organizations, helping them win a number of grants. These awards included funding to develop patient-centered medical homes (PCMHs), funding from the Office of the National Coordinator for Health Information Technology to expand electronic health records (also a focus of PCMHs), and an award from the Centers for Medicare and Medicaid Services (CMS) Comprehensive Primary Care (CPC)

Initiative to develop innovative models for controlling Medicare, Medicaid, and commercial health care spending. Buoyed by this support, the collaboration designed and implemented a comprehensive intervention, the Healthy Communities Initiative, to improve health care delivery in the Cincinnati metropolitan area.

The Intervention

The overarching goal of the Healthy Communities Initiative was based on the Institute for Healthcare Improvement's (IHI's) "Triple Aim," which calls for (1) improving the health of populations, (2) improving the patient experience of care, and (3) reducing the cost of care. Such an approach targets all levels of the health system and reflects the complex nature of the current health care environment. The stakeholders for the initiative included large employers, health plans, health systems and providers, and community and government organizations.

To achieve the Triple Aim, the stakeholders focused on five strategic priorities:

- **coordinated primary care** focused on transforming local practices into PCMHs, a health care delivery model with the goal of delivering comprehensive, coordinated, patient-centered, accessible care with an emphasis on evidence-based quality and safety
- **health information exchanges** to support communication, clinical decisionmaking, and coordinated care by making individual patient information available to a wide range of health service providers
- **quality improvement** focused on two common chronic conditions: childhood asthma and adult type II diabetes (Both of these conditions, prevalent in the Cincinnati population, can be controlled through evidence-based processes in ambulatory settings. Failure to follow those standards can lead to costly exacerbations, as well as avoidable ED use and hospitalizations, also called ambulatory care sensitive admissions.)
- **public reporting and consumer engagement** through a website to publicly report quality measures, which is thought to improve care quality by empowering patients to choose higher-quality care providers and, in turn, spurring providers to improve care delivery
- **payment innovations** to create aligned incentives for providers, patients, and health plans so that they follow best practices and use resources prudently.

The Evaluation

We conducted a rigorous evaluation of the initiative's impact during its first three years. The goal of our analysis was to assess the effect of the Healthy Communities Initiatives in Cincinnati on the Triple Aim of better health, better care, and lower cost for the first three years of this ongoing intervention.

We utilized three sources of public and private data to compare health and behavioral risk factors, employment status, and health care utilization for the Cincinnati metropolitan area with 15 other major metropolitan statistical areas (MSAs) with similarly sized populations.[1] Measures for the "better health" dimension were derived from the Selected Metropolitan Area Risk Trends (SMART) data of the Behavioral Risk Factor Surveillance System (BRFSS), which contain information on health risk factors including obesity, smoking, and alcohol consumption (Centers for Disease Control and Prevention, 2012), and the Current Population Survey (CPS), which has data on time missed from work due to illness (U.S. Census Bureau and the Bureau of Labor Statistics, 2012).

To measure outcomes related to the "better care" dimension of the Triple Aim, we used measures from two sources: the Healthcare Effectiveness Data and Information Set (HEDIS), which is used to benchmark health plans and is maintained by the National Committee for Quality Assurance (NCQA), an agency that accredits health plans; and the Prevention Quality Indicators developed by the Agency for Healthcare Research and Quality (AHRQ), an agency of the U.S. Department of Health and Human Services. Both used the Truven MarketScan Research Database, a national database of health plan claims.

To measure outcomes related to the "lower costs" dimension, we examined health care costs on a per-member-per-month (PMPM) basis drawing from inpatient, outpatient, ED, and prescription drug claims in the MarketScan database.

Our analysis estimated the differential changes in our measures between Cincinnati and the reference cities during the first three intervention years (2010–2012) compared with a baseline period of 2006–2009. We controlled for individual- and market-level factors to make the reference cities and their residents comparable to the Cincinnati market.

Summary of Findings

Compared to the 15 reference cities, Cincinnati residents were more likely to be non-Hispanic white, less likely to have completed college, and more likely to participate in a high-deductible health plan (HDHP). At baseline, Cincinnati residents had a smaller number of hours missed from work due to illness in the last week, a lower self-reported health status, more office-based primary care visits, more ED visits, more prescription drug fills, and larger total health care costs, and were more likely to be obese and to binge drink. However, the prevalence of chronic conditions among Cincinnati residents was similar to the prevalence among residents in the reference cities. The remainder of this section summarizes the most salient findings. The findings are summarized in Table S.1.

BETTER HEALTH

The Healthy Communities Initiative in Cincinnati was associated with improved employee productivity. Over the course of the intervention, the percentage of people in Cincinnati who responded

[1] The 15 MSAs include Charlotte-Gastonia-Rock Hill, N.C.-S.C.; Cleveland-Elyria-Mentor, Ohio; Columbus, Ohio; Denver-Aurora-Broomfield, Col.; Jacksonville, FL; Kansas City, Mo.-Kan.; Las Vegas-Paradise, Nev.; Memphis, Tenn.-Miss.-Ark.; Nashville-Davidson-Murfreesboro-Franklin, Tenn.; Orlando-Kissimmee-Sanford, Fla.; Portland-Vancouver-Hillsboro, Ore.-Wash.; Providence-New Bedford-Fall River, R.I.-Mass.; San Antonio-New Braunfels, Texas; San Jose-Sunnyvale-Santa Clara, Calif.; and St. Louis, Mo.-Ill.

Executive Summary

Table S.1. Intervention Effects on Health, Quality of Care, Health Care Utilization, and Health Care Cost

Domain	Outcome Metrics	Intervention Years		
		2010	2011	2012
Health	Self-reported health status	—	—	—
	Obesity	—	—	—
	Smoking	—	—	—
	Binge drinking	—	—	—
Productivity	Any missed work due to illness	—	—	↓
	Work hours missed due to illness	—	—	↓
Access to primary care	Adults' access to preventive/ambulatory health services	—	—	↓
	Children's and adolescents' access to primary care practitioners	↓	↓	↓
Chronic care	Percentage of patients using angiotensin receptor blockers (ARBs)/angiotensin-converting enzyme (ACE) inhibitors who receive appropriate monitoring	—	↓	↓
	Percentage of patients on diuretics receiving appropriate monitoring	—	↓	↓
	Percentage of asthma patients receiving appropriate medications	↓	↓	—
	Percentage of diabetic patients receiving hemoglobin A1c testing	—	↓	—
	Percentage of diabetic patients receiving low-density lipoprotein cholesterol testing	—	—	—
	Percentage of patients with lower back pain without imaging within 28 days of the diagnosis	—	—	—
Preventable admissions and ED visits	Ambulatory care sensitive inpatient admissions	—	—	↓
	Inpatient readmissions within 30 days of discharge	↓	—	—
	Potentially avoidable ED visits	—	—	—
Outpatient	Office-based primary care visits	↓	↓	↓
	Outpatient PMPM cost	—	—	—
Prescription drug	Prescription drug fills	↓	↓	↓
	Prescription drug PMPM cost	—	↓	↓
Emergency care	ED visits	↑	↑	↑
	ED PMPM cost	—	↑	—
Inpatient care	Inpatient admissions	—	—	—
	Inpatient PMPM cost	—	—	—
Total cost	Total PMPM Cost	—	—	—

NOTE: The table shows the changes in Cincinnati relative to the reference cities. — indicates no statistically significant findings.
↑ represents a statistically significant increase in Cincinnati relative to the reference cities (p≤0.05). Compared to the reference cities, an outcome metric may increase more or decline less in Cincinnati. ↓ represents a statistically significant decrease in Cincinnati relative to the reference cities (p≤0.05). Compared to the reference cities, an outcome metric may increase less or decline more in Cincinnati.

that they had missed work dropped by about 1 percentage point, while it remained almost constant in the reference cities. In 2012, we found a significant decline in the likelihood of being absent from work, which translated to an estimated 7,281 fewer Cincinnati employees calling in sick over the course of the year. In addition, there was a trend toward a decrease in the mean number of hours missed per person per year over the course of the intervention. For 2012, the difference amounted to about 140,000 working hours or about 70 full time–equivalent (FTE) employees. Nonetheless, the intervention was not linked to significant improvements in residents' health and health behaviors.

We found improvements in preventable hospital admissions and readmissions that point to better care coordination, particularly for higher-risk patients. Ambulatory care sensitive admissions decreased from 4.73 per 1,000 residents (0.55 more than the reference cities) during the baseline period, to 3.72 per 1,000 in 2012—a significant decrease. However, we found that adherence to evidence-based recommendations for chronic care management decreased in Cincinnati compared with the reference cities.

At the same time, use of primary and outpatient care decreased in Cincinnati compared with the reference cities. During the baseline years, Cincinnati averaged 1,714 outpatient visits per 1,000 member years, about 36 visits per year more than the reference cities. The number of office-based primary care visits declined significantly in all years of the intervention, though the decline reflected fewer than five visits per 1,000 member years in 2010–2011. By 2012, we estimated that Cincinnati residents had 136 fewer office-based primary care visits per 1,000 member years than the reference cities.

During this period, use of prescription drugs decreased also. In 2009, Cincinnati residents had an estimated 5,234 prescriptions per 1,000 residents, 108 more prescriptions per year than statistically similar residents of the reference cities. By 2011, we estimated 510 fewer prescriptions per 1,000 residents in Cincinnati. In other words, a Cincinnati resident used about 0.5 fewer prescriptions per year after the second year of the intervention.

Use of ED services increased during the intervention. Utilization increased significantly in Cincinnati relative to the reference cities during the three intervention years. Cincinnati began the intervention with approximately 161 ED visits per 1,000 member years, or seven more ED visits per 1,000 member years than the reference cities. That difference rose to 13 more visits per 1,000 member years by 2011 before dropping to only ten more visits in 2012. The differences between Cincinnati and the reference cities changed significantly from the baseline difference during the intervention years.

LOWER COST

Among the changes in utilization patterns, only the change in prescription drug use led to lower prescription costs, but no statistically significant changes in overall health care costs were observed.

Discussion

BETTER HEALTH

The absence of a strong effect of the intervention on health status indicators, such as body weight and smoking rates, is not surprising. First, it may take more than three years to observe significant changes in health behaviors and status. In addition, the intervention did not explicitly target health-related behaviors; rather, it largely focused on improving medical care. Even well-resourced and personalized interventions, such as workplace wellness programs, are known to have only

Executive Summary

a limited effect on health-related behaviors, such as smoking cessation and physical activities (Mattke, Liu, et al., 2013). Thus, it is to be expected that improvements in health are unlikely to materialize as a "side effect" of the interventions. However, we found a differential decrease in illness-related work loss in Cincinnati. While instances of sick leave declined in both Cincinnati and the 15 reference markets after 2009 (presumably as a consequence of the recession), the trend was much stronger in Cincinnati and the difference reached statistical significance in 2012, the third year of the intervention. Because the trend is adjusted for differences in age structure and burden of disease between Cincinnati and the reference markets, we interpret it as an early sign of improved health of the workforce.

BETTER CARE

We found that the Healthy Communities Initiative in Cincinnati was significantly associated with reductions in hospital readmissions and ambulatory care sensitive hospital admissions, suggesting improved care coordination and better post-discharge management for higher-risk patients. During the intervention period, the Greater Cincinnati Health Council's Accountable Care Transformation group engaged 21 hospitals in reducing readmissions and improving care coordination after a hospital admission, which could contribute to the decline in hospital readmissions. Additionally, the 2012 introduction of the HealthBridge alert system is likely to have contributed to this result, as it notifies primary care providers if one of their patients has been admitted to the hospital or visited the ED, and thus facilitates planning and management of care transitions. As mentioned above, by October 2012, 87 sites were running and 26,000 alerts had been sent (U.S. Department of Health and Human Services and Office of the National Coordinator for Health Information Technology, November 2012).

At the same time, the observed decline in use of primary and outpatient care and of prescription drugs is counterintuitive, as is the lower adherence to evidence-based recommendations for chronic care management and increased ED use. If the intervention worked as expected, we would observe increased use of primary care and prescriptions, improved chronic disease management, and fewer inpatient admissions and ED visits.

It should be emphasized that a *finding of no effect* would not have been entirely surprising, as the intervention is still in its early stage. While formally in its third year at the time of the evaluation, many of the more fundamental changes are just beginning to take effect. Better access to high-quality primary care through the promulgation of the PCMH concept is one of the cornerstones of the initiative. As of mid-2013, 84 practices in the Cincinnati MSA had obtained NCQA Level 3 PCMH recognition, representing about 24 percent of the primary care providers in Cincinnati. Practices that have only recently obtained their PCMH designation may not have reached their full potential. A recent study of a medical home pilot in Pennsylvania did not detect significant effects on utilization or cost of care, and only a limited effect on quality of care over a three-year intervention (Friedberg et al., 2014). Similarly, a new alert system of the HealthBridge health information exchange was implemented in 2012.

Yet finding *opposite trends* from what we expected is surprising, although it can likely be explained by the wide adoption of HDHPs in Cincinnati relative to the reference markets during these first three years of the Healthy Communities Initiative. The share of HDHPs in Cincinnati more than doubled from 13.4 percent in 2009 to 28.5 percent in 2012, but only increased from 7.5 percent to 10.8 percent in the reference cities during the same time frame. As HDHPs shift responsibility for health care costs to plan members, they have profound impacts on utilization patterns. Prior literature suggests that HDHPs reduce health care spending by 5 to 14 percent on average, although the effect varies across employers (Bundorf, 2012). Cost savings from HDHPs are primarily because of reductions in prescription cost and outpatient cost. HDHPs have no consistent effect on inpatient admissions; they have modest to no reductions in preventive service use when they are exempted from the deductible and significant reductions when they are not. Consumers in HDHPs may indiscriminately reduce utilization.

To account for the adoption of HDHPs in our analysis, we included an indicator for HDHP in all the models and also conducted sensitivity analyses using the individuals who were always in an HDHP or never in an HDHP during 2006–2012 under the assumption that these individuals did not experience a significant change in cost-sharing arrangements and thus would not likely change their care-seeking behavior. However, the results in those subsamples were largely similar to those in the overall population. One possible explanation is that the rapid adoption of HDHPs in the Cincinnati market affected not only the individuals in HDHPs but also those not in them. This hypothesis is consistent with prior research showing that providers tend to orient their practice patterns to the average or modal insurance coverage in their catchment areas (Glied and Zivin, 2002; Hu and Reuben, 2002; Landon, 2004). A caveat, however, is that this body of literature is primarily based on the experience in managed care, which typically imposes financial incentives on providers, whereas in this case, HDHPs primarily influence patient care-seeking behaviors. It is also possible that other unobserved factors, such as new provider payment arrangements, led to the similarity in findings between individuals who never enrolled in an HDHP and those in the full sample.

LOWER COST

Changes in use of care did not translate into changes in overall cost of care during the first three years of the intervention. This finding can be explained by the fact that payment innovations—which, based on prior research, are the most likely instrument to reduce overall cost—were implemented only recently in Cincinnati. In the Cincinnati-Dayton region, 75 practices have joined the Centers for Medicaid and Medicare Services' CPC Initiative, in which payers offer bonus payments to primary care providers who effectively coordinate patient care. In addition, Cincinnati's Mercy Health System is involved in a national payment reform pilot with the CMS Medicare Shared Savings Program, but the initiative became operational only in the fall of 2012.

Limitations of the Analysis

This analysis had several limitations. First and foremost, unobservable differences between Cincinnati and the 15 reference markets, as well as their respective residents, may have influenced our results. The CPS and BRFSS data did not allow us to track individuals over time, and it might have reduced our ability to detect the intervention effect. In addition, we were not able to control for the changes in the health care delivery systems of other markets during the study period. This challenge could have led to an underestimation of the effect of the interventions implemented in Cincinnati. Further, no data were available on nontraditional forms of care delivery in PCMHs, such as phone consultations or electronic exchanges between providers and patients. It is likely that nontraditional services substitute for in-person physician visits. If this is true, office-based primary care visits are not a good measure for quality improvement resulting from PCMHs because a decrease in office-based primary care visits might not reflect an actual decline in access to primary care. Moreover, we were not able to tease out the potential selection in HDHP participation. GE, as one of the largest employers in Cincinnati, required all salaried employees to join an HDHP in 2010 and required all production employees to do the same in 2012. But we are not sure whether an HDHP plan was the only option among other employers in Cincinnati or employers in the reference cities. This potential selection bias may have confounded our sensitivity analyses for those always or never enrolled in an HDHP plan.

Conclusions

We conducted the first quantitative evaluation on the Healthy Communities Initiative in Cincinnati for its first three intervention years. Overall, our findings were largely inconclusive because of the concomitant marketwide shift to HDHPs and the early stage of the intervention.

Transitions to HDHPs are known to affect care-seeking behaviors profoundly—particularly immediately after a change in benefit design, as plan members adapt to the new incentives. As the share of HDHP plans more than doubled in Cincinnati during our analysis period, it may have concealed intervention effects. As the level of HDHP penetration in Cincinnati stabilizes—and, thus, the effect of switching to HDHPs on utilizations and costs decreases—analyzing additional years of data will allow the effect of the intervention to be disentangled from the effect of benefit design changes.

As key components of the intervention—such as payment redesign, PCMHs, and the HealthBridge alert notification—were still being fully implemented during the period of analysis, the intervention will not have been able to take full effect. We did find some encouraging signs that better care coordination bears fruit, such as less illness-related work loss and fewer avoidable hospital admissions and readmissions. These early impacts suggest that the initiative may succeed in improving care, lowering cost, and improving health status if given sufficient time. Therefore, a future evaluation of the Healthy Communities Initiative in Cincinnati will be able to assess a more mature program, leverage more data, and result in more conclusive findings.

Acknowledgments

FUNDING FOR THIS PROJECT WAS PROVIDED BY THE GENERAL ELECTRIC CORPORATION (GE). WE would like to thank GE for their guidance and feedback throughout the development of this report. In particular, we are grateful to Adam Malinoski, Alan Gilbert, and Craig Osterhues who gave generously of their time to review this report and share background knowledge on the Cincinnati health care context.

Many staff members at RAND helped us develop this evaluation. We thank Bing Han for providing statistical guidance, Teague Ruder for preparing the data sets and performing many of the analyses, Carole Gresenz for her valuable input into the evaluation design and interpretation of results, and Clare Stevens and Patrick Orr for their overall support of the project team in the publication of this report.

We would also like to thank Drs. Janice Blanchard and David Auerbach for their careful review of this report.

Acknowledgments

Abbreviations

ACE	angiotensin-converting enzyme
AHRQ	Agency for Healthcare Research and Quality
ARB	angiotensin receptor blockers
BLS	Bureau of Labor Statistics
BMI	body mass index
BRFSS	Behavioral Risk Factor Surveillance System
CDC	Centers for Disease Control and Prevention
CMS	Centers for Medicare and Medicaid Services
CPC	Comprehensive Primary Care
CPS	Current Population Survey
CT	computerized tomography
ED	emergency department
HbA1C	hemoglobin A1c
HER	electronic health record
FTE	full time–equivalent
GE	General Electric
HDHP	high-deductible health plan
HEDIS	Healthcare Effectiveness Data and Information Set
HIE	health information exchange
IHI	Institute for Healthcare Improvement
LDL-c	low-density lipoprotein cholesterol
MRI	magnetic resonance imaging
MSA	metropolitan statistical area
NCQA	National Committee for Quality Assurance
PCMH	patient-centered medical home
PMPM	per member per month
PQI	Prevention Quality Indicators
SMART	Selected Metropolitan Area Risk Trends

Abbreviations

Introduction

Background to the Project

Metropolitan Cincinnati residents have traditionally had among the highest health care costs in the United States, yet little evidence exists that people are getting their money's worth, especially in terms of preventive and primary care. On measures of overuse of care—such as emergency department (ED) visits or hospital admissions for ambulatory care sensitive conditions that should be managed in primary care settings, such as asthma—Cincinnati's rates are higher than state and national averages. Cincinnati also has above-average rates of preventable mortality (Radley and Commonwealth Fund, 2012).

Recognizing that high health care spending was not resulting in a healthy and productive population, community leaders began to prioritize local health care reform in 2007, long before it became a national priority. Recently, large employers, health plans, and health care providers in the Cincinnati area joined with community organizations in a renewed effort to simultaneously lower costs and increase quality. Several factors unique to Cincinnati have spurred this initiative:

- the presence of several large employers (including General Electric [GE], Procter and Gamble, and The Kroger Co.) desiring to keep their employees healthy while controlling their health care costs
- changes to the health care infrastructure, including the consolidation of some hospitals and health care systems, resulting in a reduction in the number of players
- a long history of actively convening organizations comprising the business and health care communities (exemplified by the Health Collaborative, the Greater Cincinnati Health Council, and HealthBridge, which combined in 2012).

In 2009, GE's Healthy Communities Initiative in Cincinnati built on and revitalized this successful collaboration among employers, health plans, providers, and community organizations, helping them win two large grants and a number of smaller ones. These awards included funding to develop patient-centered medical homes (PCMHs), funding from the Office of the National Coordinator for Health Information Technology to expand electronic health records (also a focus of PCMHs), and an award from the Centers for Medicare and Medicaid Services (CMS) Comprehensive Primary Care (CPC) Initiative to develop innovative models for controlling Medicare, Medicaid, and commercial health care spending. Buoyed by this support, the collaboration designed and implemented a comprehensive intervention to improve health care delivery in the Cincinnati metropolitan area.

The Intervention

The overarching goal of the Healthy Communities Initiative was based on the Institute for Healthcare Improvement's (IHI) "Triple Aim," which calls for (1) improving the patient experience of care, (2) improving the health of populations, and (3) reducing the per capita cost of care (IHI, 2013). Such an approach targets all levels of the health system and reflects the complex nature of the current health care environment. The stakeholders for the initiative included large employers, health plans, health systems and providers, and community and government organizations.[1] To achieve the Triple Aim, the stakeholders focused on five strategic priorities:

- coordinated primary care
- health information exchanges (HIEs)
- quality improvement
- public reporting and consumer engagement
- payment innovations.

We discuss each of these priorities in more detail below.

Coordinated Primary Care. To achieve the goal of improving primary care coordination, the stakeholders focused on transforming local medical practices into PCMHs, a health care delivery model with the goal of delivering comprehensive, coordinated, patient-centered, accessible care with an emphasis on evidence-based quality and safety. Practices wishing to adopt the PCMH model were permitted to implement some or all of these components and in varying degrees. Although evaluations of the PCMH model have reported varying effects, recent systematic reviews found that, overall, PCMHs improve quality of care, reduce errors, improve patient experience, and reduce ED visits in older patients (Rosenthal, 2008; Jackson et al., 2013). Toward that end, the Health Collaborative received an Aligning Forces for Quality grant from the Robert Wood Johnson Foundation in 2007 to provide seed money to ten PCMH pilot practices. In 2010, the Health Collaborative received $4.2 million from Bethesda Inc. to fund additional PCMH transitions (Mattke et al., 2013b).

---

[1] Examples of stakeholders (Mattke et al., 2013b) include the following:
- Employers: Ethicon Endo-Surgery, Inc.; GE Aviation; The Kroger Co.; Macy's, Inc.; Procter and Gamble
- Health plans: Anthem Blue Cross Blue Shield
- Health systems and providers: Cincinnati Children's Hospital; Mercy Health; St. Elizabeth Healthcare; TriHealth
- Community and government organizations: Hamilton County Public Health, HealthBridge, The Greater Cincinnati Health Council, The Health Collaborative.

As of mid-2013, 84 practices in the Cincinnati metropolitan statistical area (MSA) had obtained Level-3 PCMH recognition from the National Committee for Quality Assurance (NCQA),[2] which represents about 24 percent of the primary care providers in the Cincinnati metropolitan area.[3] Practices that have only recently obtained their PCMH designation are still in the nascent stage of transformation, and may not have reached their full potential (Friedberg et al., 2014).

HIEs. Effective HIEs support communication, clinical decisionmaking, and coordinated care by making individual patient information available to a wide range of health service providers. By aggregating data, HIEs allow health systems to evaluate their own practices and use this information to improve clinical processes and outcomes. HealthBridge received a federal grant to establish a center to support practices as they implement and achieve "meaningful use" of electronic health records. During the intervention period, Cincinnati went from roughly 30 percent to more than 60 percent of physicians using electronic health records.

The HealthBridge health information exchange has been electronically delivering clinical data across the market for more than 12 years, and currently receives approximately five million results per month. At the time of the evaluation, a new functionality implemented in 2012 was an alert system that notified providers if one of their patients had been admitted to a hospital or emergency room. By October 2012, 87 sites were running and 26,000 alerts had been sent (U.S. Department of Health and Human Services and Office of the National Coordinator for Health Information Technology, November 2012).

Quality Improvement. Cincinnati's improvement efforts focused on two critical chronic conditions: childhood asthma and adult type II diabetes. For example, to improve quality in the treatment of childhood asthma, Cincinnati Children's hospital created an asthma registry to track high-risk patients for targeted outreach. Some practices also utilized asthma care coordinators and electronic health records to track high-quality care (Mattke et al., 2013b). For adult type II diabetes, the alert system mentioned above was utilized for diabetics accessing ED services for diabetes-related care—and some practices began tracking a composite measure of diabetes quality indicators (Mattke, Sorbero, et al., 2013). Both of these conditions, prevalent in the Cincinnati population, can be controlled through evidence-based processes in ambulatory settings; failure to follow those standards can lead to costly exacerbations, as well as avoidable ED use and hospitalizations.

Public Reporting and Consumer Engagement. Meaningful improvements in health care cannot happen without patient involvement. Recognizing this, the stakeholders set out to engage and inform health care consumers by developing a website to publicly report quality measures, with the intention of improving care quality by empowering patients to choose higher-quality care providers and, in turn, spurring providers to improve care delivery (Hibbard, Stockard, and Tusler, 2005).

Payment Innovations. Payment innovation seeks to create aligned incentives for providers, patients, and health plans so that they follow best practices and use resources prudently. The CPC

---

[2] NCQA Level-3 PCMH recognition is awarded to practices that score between 85 and 100 points on the NCQA's six PCMH standards and have a 50-percent performance level or higher on six "must pass" items (see Appendix A, Table A.3, available online).

[3] According to the data on the NCQA website, there are 397 individual physicians in the 84 certified PCMH practices that have achieved Level 3 recognition from the NCQA out of a total of 1,653 primary care physicians (including pediatricians) in the Cincinnati MSA, based on data from the 2012 Area Resource File.

Initiative, through which Medicare and private payers offer bonus payments to providers for effective care coordination, has a dual goal of cost savings and improved primary care. At the time of the evaluation, however, only 75 practices in the Cincinnati-Dayton region had joined the CPC Initiative (Mattke et al., 2013b).

The Evaluation

In this report, we summarize the results from a rigorous quantitative evaluation of the Healthy Communities Initiative using three sources of public and private data to compare health and behavioral risk factors, employment status, and health care utilization for the Cincinnati MSA to 15 other MSAs with similarly sized populations (see Table A.1 in Appendix A, available online, for details). Measures for better health were derived from the Selected Metropolitan Area Risk Trends (SMART) data of the Behavioral Risk Factor Surveillance System (BRFSS), which contain information on health behaviors including obesity, smoking, and alcohol consumption, and the Current Population Survey (CPS), which has data on time missed from work due to illness. Measures for better care and lower costs were constructed from the Truven MarketScan data, a national database of health insurance claims.

Data and Methods

To evaluate the impact of the Healthy Communities Initiative on the Triple Aim of better health, better care, and lower costs, we aimed to estimate the differential changes in measures by comparing trend data reflecting the Triple Aim from the Cincinnati MSA to those for 15 other MSAs with similarly sized populations (see Table A.1 in Appendix A, available online, for details). This approach allowed us to separate the effect of the Healthy Communities Initiative from the secular time trends in various outcomes. Measures for better health were derived from the SMART data of the BRFSS and the CPS. We describe these data in greater detail next. Measures for better care and lower costs were constructed from the MarketScan Research Database, a national database of commercial health insurance claims. The comparison MSAs were selected based on their population size and the availability of data in the MarketScan Research Database. According to the 2012 CPS data, as illustrated in Figure 2.1, the Cincinnati MSA had a population of 2.13 million, whereas the average population size of the 15 comparison MSAs was 1.97 million, ranging from 1.25 million to 2.82 million. The comparison states cover 20 states, including Ohio.

Data Sources

As summarized in Table 2.1, we used three different data sources to examine whether the intervention had an effect on health, health care, and cost. We describe each data source in detail.

BEHAVIORAL RISK FACTOR SURVEILLANCE SYSTEM

BRFSS is an annual survey conducted by the Centers for Disease Control and Prevention (CDC). It is based on an annual, cross-sectional probability sample of the U.S. adult population using landline telephone and, after 2010, cell phone numbers. Individuals are interviewed over the phone about their health-related behaviors that cause morbidity and mortality among the U.S. adult population, including smoking, alcohol use, physical activity, diet, hypertension, and safety belt use. The survey also collects sociodemographic information. For the purpose of this project, we used the SMART BRFSS data files (CDC, 2012). These files were derived by the CDC and allow users

Figure 2.1. Location and Population Sizes of Cincinnati and 15 Reference Markets

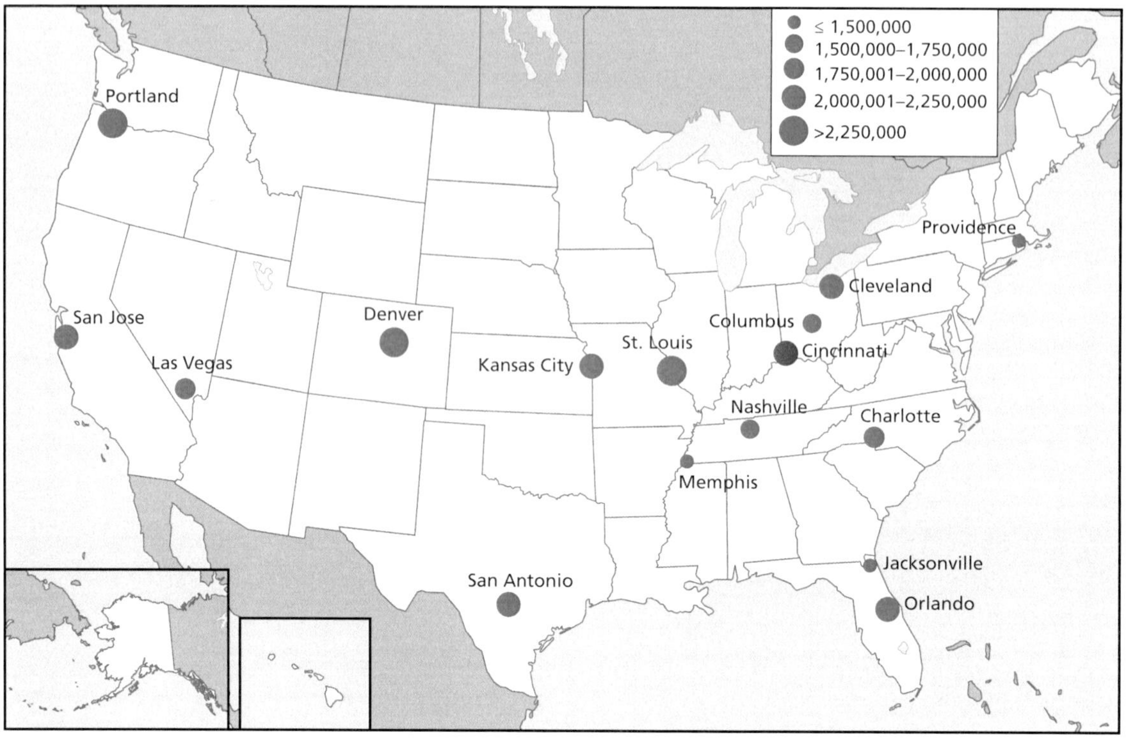

Legend:
- ● ≤ 1,500,000
- ● 1,500,000–1,750,000
- ● 1,750,001–2,000,000
- ● 2,000,001–2,250,000
- ● >2,250,000

SOURCE: Authors' analysis of CPS data, 2012.
RAND *RR729-2.1*

to estimate the prevalence rates specifically for various MSAs with more than 500 respondents in the annual BRFSS sample.

CURRENT POPULATION SURVEY

The CPS collects annual, nationally representative data on individual and household characteristics, labor force status, and employment characteristics. It is administered by the U.S. Census Bureau and the Bureau of Labor Statistics (BLS) and surveys a sample of approximately 60,000 noninstitutional and occupied U.S. households each month, covering all 50 states and the District of Columbia (U.S. Census Bureau and BLS, 2012). All individuals within a sampled household are eligible for participation in the CPS survey as long as they meet the age criterion (15 years and older) and are not actively serving in the U.S. armed forces. However, information on labor force status and employment characteristics are only collected for individuals older than 16. Each household is interviewed once a month for four consecutive months, left out for eight months, then interviewed again once a month for four consecutive months before it is retired permanently from the CPS sample.

MARKETSCAN RESEARCH DATABASE

We examined trends between 2006 and 2012 in measures for better care and lower cost using a commercially available claims database called the Truven Health MarketScan® Research Databases (Truven Health Analytics, 2012). The MarketScan Research Database provides a nationally generalizable sample of the commercially insured population. It is widely used for longitudinal and comparative analyses of treatment patterns and costs of care, and it contains more than 500 million medical and drug claims from approximately 100 payers. The database has inpatient admission records, outpatient services, prescriptions, and allowed charges for services. The medical claims allow users to see which services a health plan member received, for which diagnoses, at which place of service, and by which type of provider. Prescription drug claims reflect active ingredient, quantity dispensed, and days supplied. All claims have information on allowed charges, as well as patient cost-sharing.

In addition to the claims, the database has documentation on the health plan members, such as age, gender, type of insurance plan, period of plan eligibility, and residence (3-digit ZIP code). All data have an anonymized individual identifier that permits tracking members over time and across places of service.

An MSA-level identifier allowed us to attribute each member to the Cincinnati MSA or to the comparison MSAs mentioned above. For the current analysis, we used data for people under 65, the age at which most people become eligible for Medicare.

Outcome Measures

BETTER HEALTH

We included the following health outcome measures in our analyses (Table 2.1):

- self-rated health status
- smoking
- obesity
- binge drinking
- missed work due to illness
- hours of missed work due to illness.

For analytic purposes, all outcomes except hours of missed work are dichotomous. Self-reported health status is reported as good or poor: Good represents those who rated their health as good, very good, or excellent; poor represents those who rated their health as poor or fair. Smoking status is reported as yes for those who indicated they were current smokers and no for all others. Individuals were reported as obese if their calculated body mass index (BMI) was greater than 30 and as not obese otherwise.[1] Binge drinking is reported as yes for those who reported at least one binge drinking event (occasions when men have five or more drinks or women have four or more drinks) during the survey year and no otherwise. Missed work due to illness is measured as yes if the CPS respondent missed work in the last week due to illness or injury. Hours missed due to illness is a continuous variable derived by subtracting the respondent's number of hours worked the previous week from the usual number of hours worked per week if the respondent reported

---

[1] BMI is a ratio of body weight (in kilograms) over squared height (in meters).

Data and Methods

Table 2.1. Measures and Data Sources for the Healthy Communities Initiative Impact Evaluation

Domain	Metrics	Data Source	Data Description
Better health	Self-reported health status	2006–2012 SMART BRFSS	An annual telephone-based survey conducted by the CDC on health status and health-related behaviors such as smoking and alcohol use
	Obesity (BMI>30)		
	Smoking		
	Binge drinking		
	Missed work due to illness Work hours missed due to illness	2006–2012 CPS	A household survey conducted by the BLS on household characteristics and employment characteristics
Better care	Percentage of adult diabetic patients receiving appropriate care for diabetes	2006–2012 MarketScan	Medical and prescription drug claims for a commercially insured population
	Percentage of child asthma patients receiving appropriate care for asthma		
	Percentage of patients using ARBs, ACE inhibitors, or diuretics who receive appropriate monitoring		
	Inpatient admissions for ambulatory care sensitive conditions per 1,000 adult member years		
	Potentially avoidable emergency room care per 1,000 adult member years		
	Percentage of hospitalized patients who are readmitted during the 30 days after discharge		
	Percentage of patients with a primary diagnosis of low back pain who did not have an imaging study (plain X-ray, MRI, CT scan) within 28 days of the diagnosis		
	Utilization for major service categories per 1,000 member years		
Lower cost	Total PMPM health care costs		
	PMPM cost and utilization per 1,000 member years for major service categories (inpatient, outpatient, emergency room, prescription drug)		

NOTE: ACE: angiotensin-converting enzyme; ARB: angiotensin receptor blockers; BMI: body mass index; PMPM: per member per month; MRI: magnetic resonance imaging; CT: computerized tomography.

missing work due to illness. Respondents who reported not being employed (e.g., unemployed, retired, <15 years old) or not having a usual number of hours worked per week were excluded from the analysis.

BETTER CARE

We used nationally accepted measures for the better care dimension of the Triple Aim to ensure credibility and comparability of findings (Table 2.1). The measures came from two sources:

- The Healthcare Effectiveness Data and Information Set (HEDIS), a set of measures for benchmarking health plans that is maintained by the NCQA, which accredits health plans
- The Prevention Quality Indicators (PQI) developed by the Agency for Healthcare Research and Quality (AHRQ), an agency of the U.S. Department of Health and Human Services.

Data and Methods

The measures for better care were derived from the MarketScan Research Database. Two HEDIS measures reflect how well patients can access care: adults' access to ambulatory and preventive care services, and children's and adolescents' access to primary care. The adult measure is the percentage of adults, age 20 and older, who received preventive care or had an ambulatory care visit in the measurement year. The children's and adolescents' measure is the percentage of children ages 12 months to 19 years with a primary care visit in the measurement year.

Quality of care metrics include HEDIS measures (NCQA, 2011) of appropriate care for

■ **Children with asthma.** This refers to the percentage of children, ages 5 to 20, diagnosed with asthma who are prescribed asthma management medication and remain on asthma medication for more than 50 percent of the days from their diagnosis until the end of the measurement year.

■ **Adult diabetics.** This includes two outcomes measures: the percentage of diabetic patients, ages 18–75, who had a low-density lipoprotein cholesterol (LDL-c) screening test; and the percentage of diabetic patients, ages 18–75, who had a test for hemoglobin A1c (HbA1c).

■ **Treatment of low back pain.** This uses the percentage of patients with a primary diagnosis of low back pain who did not have an imaging study (X-ray, MRI, CT scan) within 28 days of the diagnosis as an indicator for avoiding overuse of diagnostic procedures.

■ **Medication monitoring for patients on ARBs, ACE inhibitors, or diuretics.** This refers to the percentage of patients who receive drug-appropriate testing and are on ARBs, ACE inhibitors, or diuretics.

The metrics also include three AHRQ PQI measures (AHRQ Quality Indicators, 2001):

■ the number of inpatient admissions for ambulatory care sensitive conditions per 1,000 adult member years

■ potentially avoidable ED care per 1,000 adult member years

■ the percentage of hospital inpatients readmitted within 30 days after discharge.

Ambulatory care sensitive hospitalization rates were based on the 16 AHRQ PQI conditions. Avoidable ED visit rates were based on a subset of 14 of those conditions, excluding two inpatient surgeries that would never be performed in an ED (see Table A. 2 in Appendix A, available online, for details).

LOWER COST

We examined health care costs on a PMPM basis, drawing from inpatient, outpatient, ED, and prescription drug claims in the MarketScan Research Database (Table 2.1). We adjusted all cost measures for inflation to 2013 dollars. Measures of health care utilization include hospital admissions per 1,000 member years, office-based primary care visits per 1,000 member years, ED visits per 1,000 member years, and drug prescriptions filled per 1,000 member years.

Data and Methods

Analytic Approach

The goal of our analysis was to assess the effect of the Healthy Communities Initiative in Cincinnati on health, health care quality, access, and utilization and costs for the first three years of this ongoing intervention. The analysis is based on a comparison of Cincinnati residents to the residents of 15 other similarly sized communities on each of the outcome measures described. Our analysis estimated the differential changes in our measures between Cincinnati and the reference cities during the first three intervention years (2010–2012) compared with a baseline period of 2006–2009. We controlled for individual- and market-level factors to make the reference cities and their residents comparable to the Cincinnati market. However, a change in employee health benefits occurred on a large scale in Cincinnati simultaneous to the intervention, which made it difficult to identify which change led to which impacts in the market. We used a significance level of 5 percent when interpreting the analysis results.

DESCRIPTIVE ANALYSES

Descriptive analyses were conducted to summarize the demographics of the Cincinnati and reference cities and to identify unadjusted trends in the data. These analyses included frequency, mean, median, and range calculations. Bivariate comparisons of demographic characteristics between Cincinnati and the reference cities were conducted to inform our statistical models.

STATISTICAL ANALYSES

All the modeling techniques were used to remove as much variation in the data that was not attributable to the intervention as possible so that identified changes could be attributed to the intervention. Our statistical approach was similar for all three datasets, attempting to identify differential impacts on our outcome measures in Cincinnati relative to the reference cities in the intervention years. The reference cities were selected because they were approximately the same size as Cincinnati, but, because the intervention and control groups were not randomized, we needed to address the demographic differences between Cincinnati and our reference cities. Mostly this was done in the models by including patient-level covariates such as age, gender, race, ethnicity, family income, marital status, employment classification, education level, number of children in the household, type of insurance coverage, and flags for chronic conditions that likely contribute to outcome measures, such as diabetes, chronic obstructive pulmonary disease, and cardiovascular disease. Specific individual-level covariates used in the models differ depending on the dataset used (BRFSS, CPS, and MarketScan) (see Appendix Section A1, available online, for a detailed description of the models). In addition, a set of calendar-year indicators was used to capture the secular trends in outcome measures. We also included a flag for each city in the models, called fixed effects, which should account for any remaining time-invariant variation among the reference cities themselves and between the reference cities and Cincinnati.

Additionally, because MarketScan data allowed us to track the same individual over time, we adopted a slightly different approach to estimate the intervention effect. The idea is to follow a cohort of individuals from the preintervention period to the intervention period and compare the differential changes in measures over time and between Cincinnati residents and those in the reference cities. Therefore, we required all individuals in the final sample to have at least one year of data both in the preintervention and intervention periods. We generated the predicted likelihood of an individual being in Cincinnati or other cities based on individual level characteristics in the pre-intervention period (2006–2009). The main model, based on MarketScan data, was weighted using the predicted likelihood, which ensured that the characteristics of residents in Cincinnati and other cities are balanced during the preintervention period in a statistical sense.

SENSITIVITY ANALYSES

Concurrent with the roll-out of the Healthy Communities Initiative, the Cincinnati market experienced a substantial increase in the number of residents with high-deductible health plans (HDHPs) relative to our reference markets (Figure 2.2). Between 2009 and 2012, the percentage of residents covered by such plans more than doubled in Cincinnati, from 13.4 percent to 28.5 percent, but it only increased from 7.5 to 10.8 percent in the reference markets. HDHPs shift financial responsibility toward consumers/patients and are known to have a strong effect on health care utilization patterns. Thus, there is a distinct possibility that this shift clouds the effect of the intervention.

While we controlled for type of insurance plan (preferred provider organization, point of service, HDHP, and other) in our statistical analysis, we also conducted separate analyses for residents that were always in an HDHP and for those who were never in such plans. Our assumption is that focusing on the residents who were always or never enrolled in an HDHP—and, therefore, whose incentives to seek care was not likely to change during the intervention period—would give us a better representation of the true intervention effect. HDHPs were identified using the type of insurance plan variable available in the MarketScan data.

Figure 2.2. Prevalence of HDHPs in Cincinnati Relative to Reference Markets

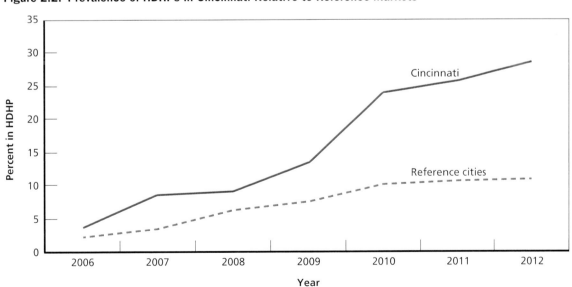

SOURCE: Authors' analysis of MarketScan data, 2006–2012.

RAND *RR729-2.2*

PRESENTATION OF THE RESULTS

To show the effects of the intervention for a general audience, we present the results using predicted outcomes based on our statistical analyses. Basically, the predicted outcome measures for a representative resident in Cincinnati are compared with those of a representative resident in the reference cities over time. A representative resident was defined as having the mean value of individual characteristics of Cincinnati residents or the residents in the reference cities.

Data and Methods

Results

Sample Descriptions

All three datasets include the data for Cincinnati and the 15 reference cities for the years 2006–2012. In the CPS data, the final sample included only individuals who were employed at the time they responded to the CPS surveys, because the measures of interest are absence from work and the number of work hours missed due to illness. This restriction resulted in a sample size of 570,019 observations (29,192 for Cincinnati and 540,827 for reference cities) for the CPS data. A final sample of 263,833 observations (12,469 for Cincinnati and 251,364 for reference cities) was provided by the SMART BRFSS data.

The final MarketScan sample included 9,619,223 observations (4,769,994 observations for the preintervention period and 4,849,229 observations for the intervention period; 791,649 for Cincinnati and 8,827,574 for the reference cities).

Compared to the reference cities, Cincinnati residents were more likely to be non-Hispanic white, less likely to have completed college, and more likely to participate in an HDHP. Unadjusted data also showed that Cincinnati residents had a smaller number of hours missed from work due to illness in the previous week, a lower self-reported health status, more office-based primary care visits, more ED visits, more prescription drug fills, larger total health care costs, and a greater likelihood of being obese and of binge drinking. However, the prevalence of chronic conditions was similar in Cincinnati residents to those in residents of the reference cities (see Tables A.6 and A.8 in Appendix A, available online).

Better Health

We did not observe a differential trend in self-reported health status, smoking behavior, obesity, and binge drinking during the first three years of the intervention, adjusting for differences in individual characteristics and those for the markets. Figure 3.1 shows that smoking rates remain about five percentage points higher in Cincinnati during the entire analysis period, and Figure 3.2 displays similar findings for obesity rates. Adjusted rates of self-reported health status and binge drinking were similar in Cincinnati and the reference markets, with no significant changes during the intervention years (see Figures A.3 and A.4 in Appendix A, available online).

Figure 3.1. Smoking Behavior in Cincinnati Relative to Reference Markets

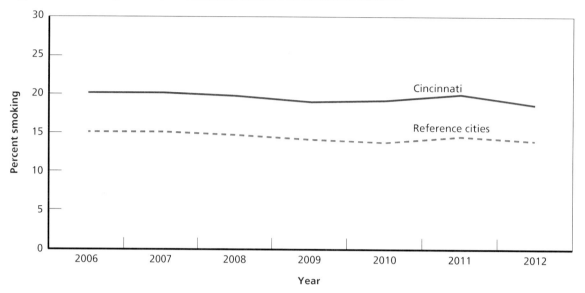

SOURCE: Authors' analysis of SMART BRFSS data, 2006–2012.
RAND *RR729-3.1*

Figure 3.2. Obesity in Cincinnati Relative to Reference Markets

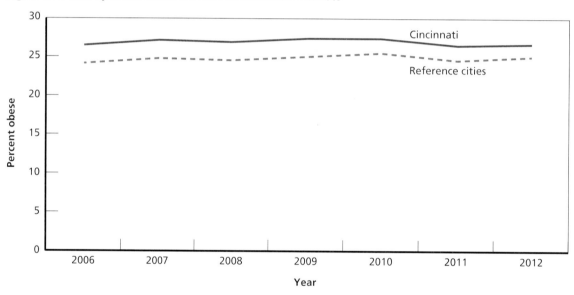

SOURCE: Authors' analysis of SMART BRFSS data, 2006–2012.
RAND *RR729-3.2*

There was a reduction in the number of people missing work in Cincinnati relative to the reference markets. At baseline, approximately 2 percent of people in Cincinnati and in the reference cities reported missing work in the last week due to illness. Over the course of the intervention, the percentage of people in Cincinnati who responded that they had missed work dropped by about 1 percentage point while it remained almost constant in the reference cities (Figure 3.3). In 2012, we found a significant decline in the likelihood of being absent from work, which translated to an estimated 7,281 fewer Cincinnati employees calling in sick over the course of the year. In addition, there was a significant difference in the mean number of hours missed per person per year over the course of the intervention (Figure 3.4). For 2012, the difference amounted to about 140,000 working hours or about 70 full time–equivalent (FTE) employees.

Figure 3.3. Percentage of Adults Who Missed Any Time at Work in the Past Week Due to Illness in Cincinnati Relative to Reference Markets

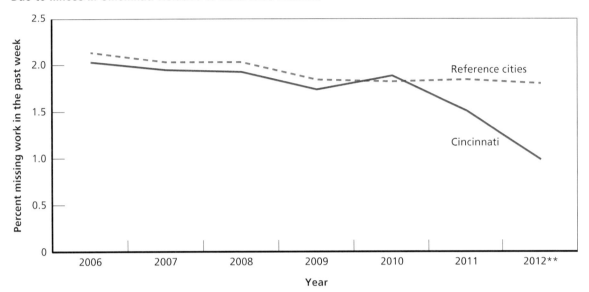

SOURCE: Authors' analysis of CPS data, 2006–2012.
NOTE: **$p \leq 0.01$ for the intervention effect.
RAND *RR729-3.3*

Figure 3.4. Mean Hours of Work Missed Due to Illness in Cincinnati Relative to Reference Markets

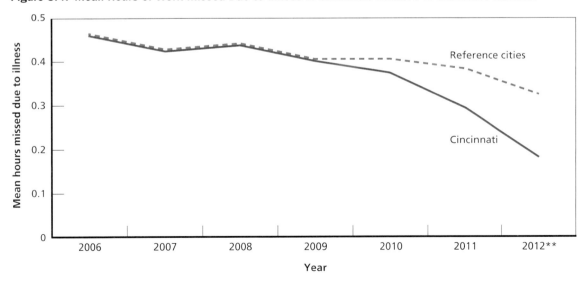

SOURCE: Authors' analysis of CPS data, 2006–2012.
NOTE: **$p \leq 0.01$ for the intervention effect.
RAND *RR729-3.4*

Results

Better Care

The results for Cincinnati show a relative decrease in access to primary care for adults and children, improvement in preventable hospital admissions and ED visits, and no improvement in the treatment of chronic conditions.

ACCESS TO PRIMARY CARE

Access to preventive/ambulatory health services increased slightly in both Cincinnati and the reference markets over the course of our analysis period. On a statistically adjusted basis, the likelihood of an adult having a preventive or ambulatory care visit increased from about 81 percent to 83 percent from 2006 to 2011. But in 2012 (the most recent intervention year for which data were available), Cincinnati gave up some of those gains, and visit rates dropped significantly, by 1 percentage point relative to the reference cities (Figure 3.5).

As Figure 3.6 shows, access to primary care for children and adolescents has historically been better in Cincinnati than in the 15 reference markets. We estimated that about 85 percent of all Cincinnati children and adolescents had a preventive or ambulatory care visit in 2006, about six percentage points more than in the reference cities. During the intervention period, children's and adolescents' access to primary care in Cincinnati remained largely unchanged, whereas that of the reference cities increased over time. The difference between Cincinnati and the reference markets decreased significantly in each year of the intervention, with Cincinnati 5.3 percentage points larger in 2010 but only 3.6 percentage points larger in 2012.

Figure 3.5. Adults' Access to Preventive/Ambulatory Health Services in Cincinnati Relative to Reference Markets

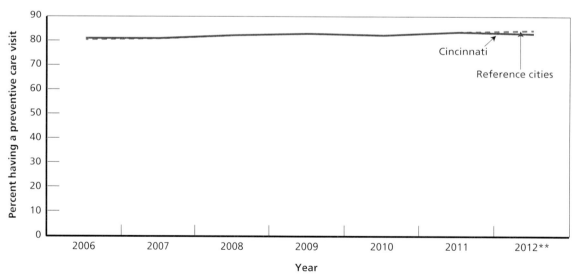

SOURCE: Authors' analysis of MarketScan data, 2006–2012.
NOTE: **p≤0.01 for the intervention effect.
RAND *RR729-3.5*

Figure 3.6. Children's and Adolescents' Access to Primary Care Practitioners

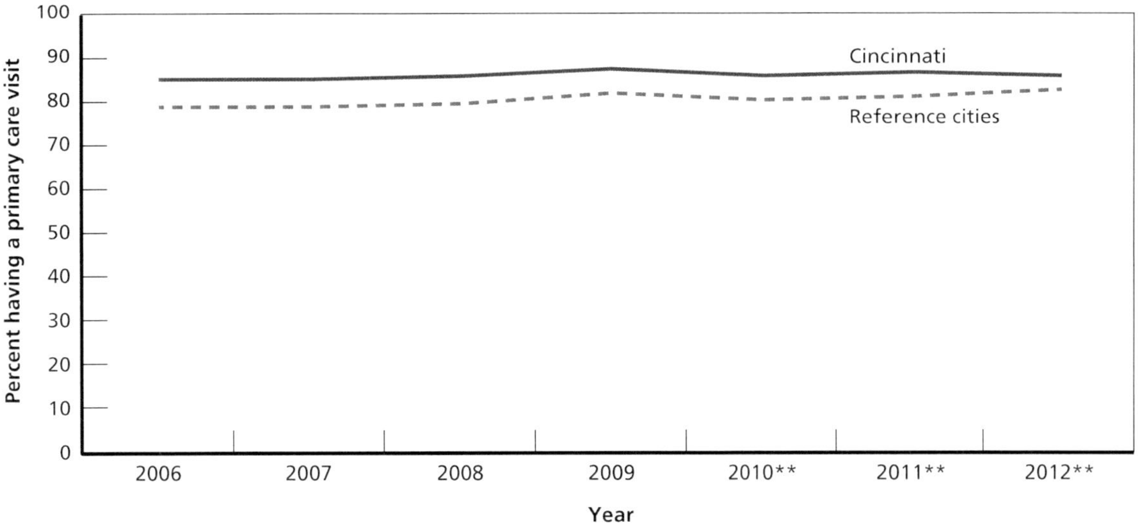

SOURCE: Authors' analysis of MarketScan data, 2006–2012.
NOTE: **p≤0.01 for the intervention effect.
RAND *RR729-3.6*

CHRONIC CARE

There was no improvement in the quality of care for chronic conditions in Cincinnati relative to the reference markets over the first three years of the intervention as measured by adherence to evidence-based treatment recommendations. Indeed, the rate at which patients on ARBs, ACE inhibitors, or diuretics were monitored with appropriate blood tests dropped significantly in 2011 and 2012 relative to the reference cities (Figures 3.7 and 3.8). At baseline, the reference cities averaged 4.5 percentage points higher in the monitoring of ARBs and ACE inhibitors and 4.1 percentage points higher in the monitoring of diuretics. In 2011, the reference cities were 6.2 percentage points higher in the monitoring of ARBs and ACE inhibitors; in 2012, 5.5 percentage points higher. Similarly, the reference cities were 6.6 percentage points higher in the monitoring of diuretics in 2011 and 5.4 percentage points higher in 2012.

As asthma and diabetes were two priorities for the intervention, we examined time trends for commonly used quality measures for those two conditions. While high overall, the rate at which asthma patients received appropriate medication declined significantly in 2010 and 2011, but then showed a nonsignificant increase in 2012 relative to the reference cities (Figure 3.9). At baseline, Cincinnati had about 1 percentage point better asthma medication use than the reference markets but the rate of appropriate use of medication for asthma in 2010 and 2011 was lower than the reference cities. The rate at which glucose control for diabetics was monitored (HbA1c testing), declined significantly in Cincinnati in 2011 but did not result in significant changes in 2010 and 2012 relative to the reference cities (Figure 3.10). While Cincinnati showed about 1 percentage point lower in glucose monitoring at baseline, it was 2.5 percentage points lower than the reference cities in 2011. Although both Cincinnati and the reference cities showed an upward trend in the rate of LDL-c testing over time, the difference in the rate of lipid testing for diabetics remained mostly unchanged over the analysis period (Figure 3.11).

Results

Figure 3.7. Percentage of Patients on ARBs or ACE Inhibitors Receiving Appropriate Monitoring in Cincinnati Relative to Reference Markets

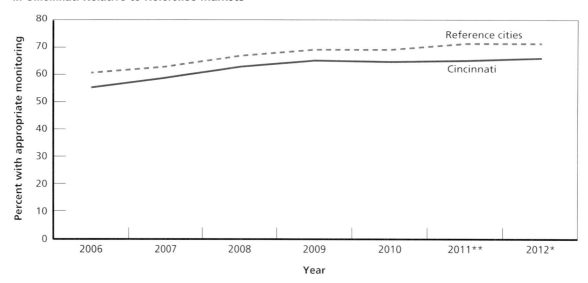

SOURCE: Authors' analysis of MarketScan data, 2006–2012.
NOTE: **p≤0.01 for the intervention effect.
RAND *RR729-3.7*

Figure 3.8. Percentage of Patients on Diuretics Receiving Appropriate Monitoring in Cincinnati Relative to Reference Markets

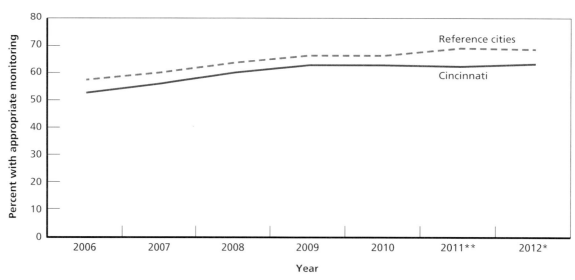

SOURCE: Authors' analysis of MarketScan data, 2006–2012.
NOTE: *p≤0.05, **p≤0.01 for the intervention effect.
RAND *RR729-3.8*

Results

Figure 3.9. Percentage of Patients with Asthma Receiving Appropriate Medications in Cincinnati Relative to Reference Markets

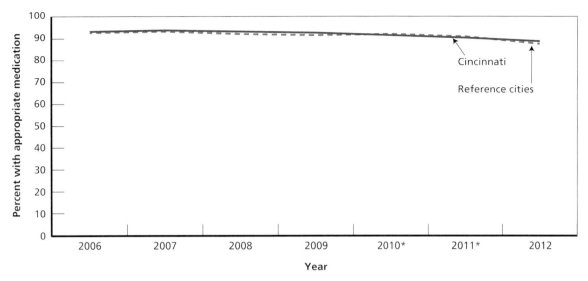

SOURCE: Authors' analysis of MarketScan data, 2006–2012.
NOTE: *p≤0.05 for the intervention effect.
RAND *RR729-3.9*

Figure 3.10. Percentage of Diabetic Patients Receiving HbA1c Testing in Cincinnati Relative to Reference Markets

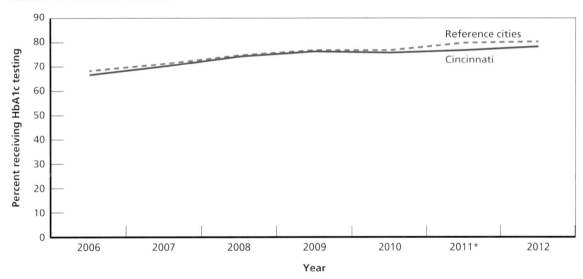

SOURCE: Authors' analysis of MarketScan data, 2006–2012.
NOTE: *p≤0.05 for the intervention effect.
RAND *RR729-3.10*

Results

Figure 3.11. Percentage of Diabetic Patients Receiving LDL-c Testing in Cincinnati Relative to Reference Markets

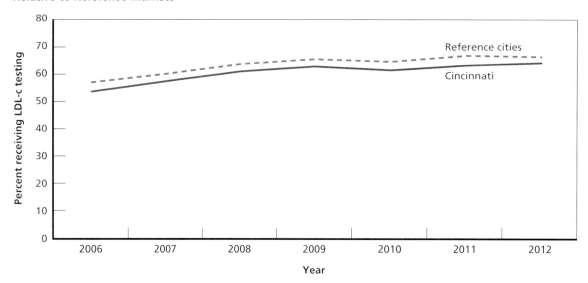

SOURCE: Authors' analysis of MarketScan data, 2006–2012.

RAND *RR729-3.11*

Figure 3.12. Percentage of Low Back Pain Patients Receiving Appropriate Care in Cincinnati Relative to Reference Markets

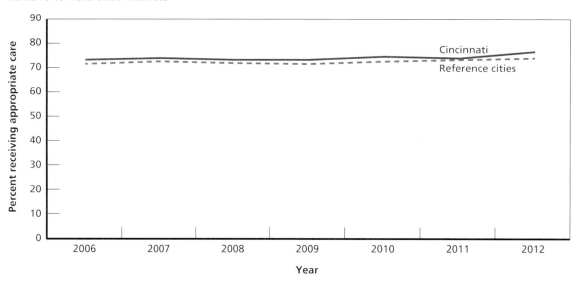

SOURCE: Authors' analysis of MarketScan data, 2006–2012.

RAND *RR729-3.12*

In the use of imaging for low back pain (an indicator of potentially inappropriate use of medical care), the difference between Cincinnati and the reference cities did not change significantly over the course of the intervention (Figure 3.12).

We found that the intervention is associated with a decrease in ambulatory sensitive care hospitalizations, as well as in readmissions within 30 days after hospital discharge, which are indicators for better access to outpatient care and improved care coordination for patients with chronic conditions.

As Figure 3.13 shows, Cincinnati averaged 4.73 ambulatory care sensitive hospital admissions per 1,000 residents, about 0.55 admissions more than in the reference cities, during the baseline period. That difference began to narrow after 2010 and, by 2012, Cincinnati's rate had dropped to 3.72 admissions per 1,000 residents fewer than the reference cities, a statistically significant change.

Similarly, readmissions to a hospital within 30 days of discharge trended downward in Cincinnati relative to the reference cities during the first three years of the intervention, and the decline in Cincinnati was statistically significant in 2010, with an estimated 0.43 fewer readmissions per 1,000 discharges (Figure 3.14). Cincinnati averaged 2.22 inpatient readmissions per 1,000 residents during the baseline period, an average of 0.03 readmissions above the reference cities. But during the intervention period, Cincinnati's readmission rate was 0.43, 0.12, and 0.18 lower than the reference cities in 2010, 2011, and 2012, respectively.

Cincinnati averaged 8.68 ED visits for ambulatory care sensitive conditions over the baseline period, 1.13 fewer visits per year than the reference cities in that period. We did not observe significant relative changes in ED use for these conditions that can typically be handled in an ambulatory care setting during the first three years of the intervention (Figure 3.15), although there was a nonsignificant increasing trend in ambulatory care sensitive ED visits in Cincinnati relative to the reference cities in 2010 and 2011 and a nonsignificant decreasing trend in 2012.

Figure 3.13. Ambulatory Care Sensitive Inpatient Admissions in Cincinnati Relative to Reference Markets

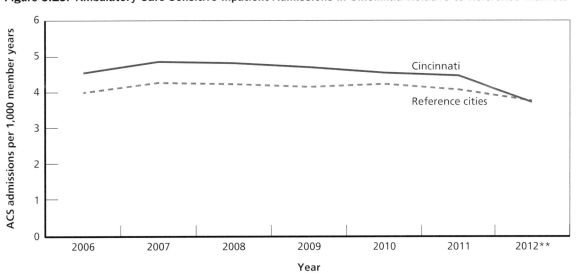

SOURCE: Authors' analysis of MarketScan data, 2006–2012.
NOTE: **p≤0.01 for the intervention effect.
RAND RR729-3.13

Results

21

Figure 3.14. Inpatient Readmissions Within 30 days of Discharge in Cincinnati Relative to Reference Markets

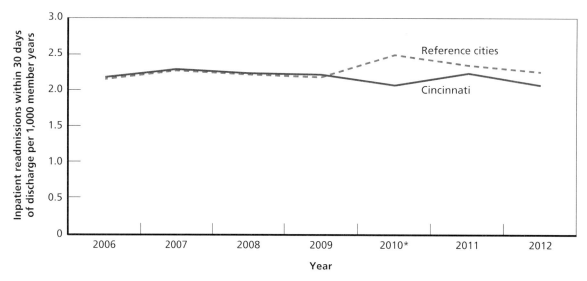

SOURCE: Authors' analysis of MarketScan data, 2006–2012.
NOTE: *p≤0.05 for the intervention effect.
RAND *RR729-3.14*

Figure 3.15. Potentially Avoidable ED Visits in Cincinnati Relative to Reference Markets

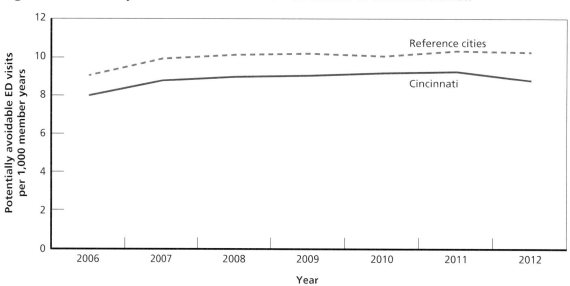

SOURCE: Authors' analysis of MarketScan data, 2006–2012.
RAND *RR729-3.15*

Results

Lower Costs

Overall, we did not detect a significant change in health care costs in Cincinnati compared with the 15 reference markets during the first three years of the intervention, but saw that utilization of outpatient care and prescription drugs declined significantly, as did prescription costs.

OUTPATIENT

On a statistically adjusted basis, we found a significant decrease in outpatient utilization in Cincinnati over the first three years of the intervention but no significant change in outpatient costs. Figures 3.16 and 3.17 show the adjusted trends in utilization and costs. During the baseline years, Cincinnati averaged 1,714 outpatient visits per 1,000 member years, about 36 visits per year more than the reference cities. The number of office-based primary care visits declined significantly in all years of the intervention, though the decline reflected fewer than five visits per 1,000 member years in 2010–2011. By 2012, we estimated that Cincinnati residents had 136 fewer office-based primary care visits per 1,000 member years than the reference cities. However, we did not observe a significant decrease in outpatient costs.

PRESCRIPTION DRUGS

Both utilization and cost of prescription drugs decreased significantly over the course of the first three intervention years. In 2009, 1,000 average Cincinnati residents had an estimated 5,234 prescriptions—and, thus, 108 more prescriptions per year than statistically similar residents of the reference cities. By 2011, we estimated 510 fewer prescriptions per 1,000 residents in Cincinnati. In other words, a Cincinnati resident used about 0.5 fewer prescriptions per year after

Figure 3.16. Office-Based Primary Care Visits in Cincinnati Relative to Reference Markets

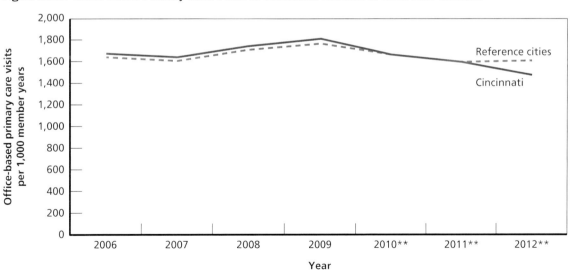

SOURCE: Authors' analysis of MarketScan data, 2006–2012.
NOTE: **p≤0.01 for the intervention effect.
RAND *RR729-3.16*

the second year of the intervention. The significant decrease in utilization in each year of the intervention translated into significant decreases in prescription costs during the intervention period (Figures 3.18 and 3.19).

EMERGENCY CARE

ED utilization increased significantly in Cincinnati during the three intervention years. Cincinnati began the intervention with approximately 161 ED visits per 1,000 member years, which was seven more ED visits per 1,000 member years than the reference cities. That difference rose

Figure 3.17. Outpatient Costs in Cincinnati Relative to Reference Markets

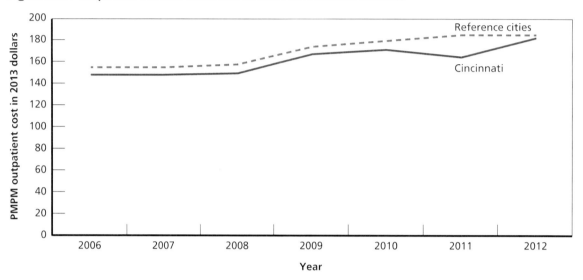

SOURCE: Authors' analysis of MarketScan data, 2006–2012.
RAND *RR729-3.17*

Figure 3.18. Prescription Drug Utilization in Cincinnati Relative to Reference Markets

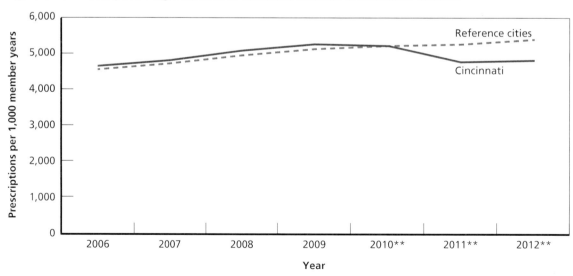

SOURCE: Authors' analysis of MarketScan data, 2006–2012.
NOTE: **p≤0.01 for the intervention effect.
RAND *RR729-3.18*

Figure 3.19. Prescription Drug Costs in Cincinnati Relative to Reference Markets

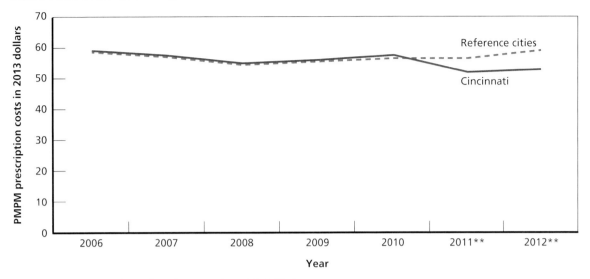

SOURCE: Authors' analysis of MarketScan data, 2006–2012.
NOTE: **p≤0.01 for the intervention effect.
RAND RR729-3.19

Figure 3.20. ED Utilization in Cincinnati Relative to Reference Markets

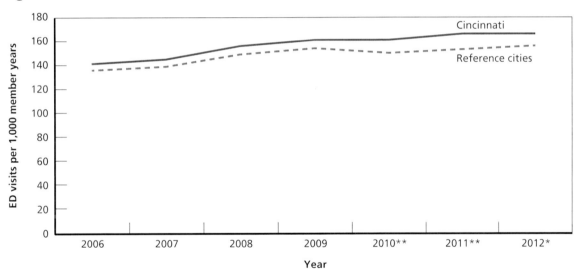

SOURCE: Authors' analysis of MarketScan data, 2006–2012.
NOTE: *p≤0.05, **p≤0.01 for the intervention effect.
RAND RR729-3.20

to 13 more visits per 1,000 member years in 2011 before dropping to ten more visits in 2012. The difference between Cincinnati and the reference cities changed significantly from the baseline difference during the intervention years (Figure 3.20). Though Cincinnati residents had more ED visits during the entire observation period, ED costs were approximately $4 PMPM lower. The difference in ED costs between the two groups decreased significantly in 2011, to $3.26, compared with the difference in preintervention years (Figure 3.21), which represents an increase in ED costs in Cincinnati relative to the reference cities in that year.

Results

Figure 3.21. ED Costs in Cincinnati Relative to Reference Markets

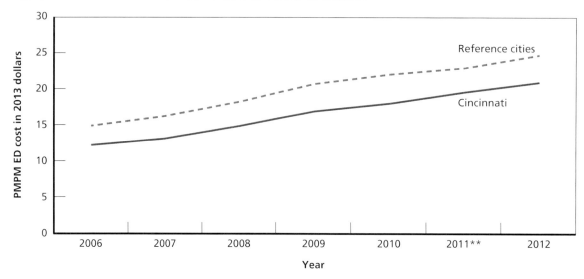

SOURCE: Authors' analysis of MarketScan data, 2006–2012.
NOTE: **p≤0.01 for the intervention effect.
RAND *RR729-3.21*

Figure 3.22. Inpatient Utilization in Cincinnati Relative to Reference Markets

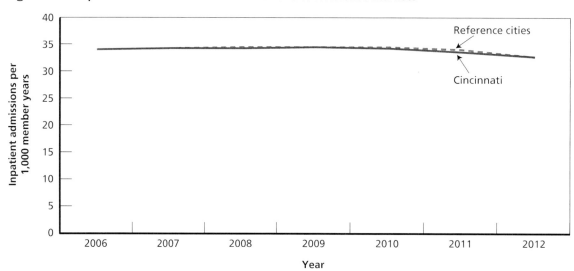

SOURCE: Authors' analysis of MarketScan data, 2006–2012.
RAND *RR729-3.22*

INPATIENT CARE

Inpatient utilization and costs were not significantly affected by the intervention. Hospital admission rates decreased slightly for both Cincinnati and the reference markets, and spending on inpatient care increased, but neither difference was statistically significant (Figures 3.22 and 3.23).

Taken together, the small changes in utilization patterns did not translate into a change in over-all spending on health care in the first three years of the Healthy Communities Initiative. In Cincinnati, as in the reference cities, costs trended upward from 2006 to 2012, with only a non-significant drop in Cincinnati in 2011, from $327 PMPM in 2010 to $319 PMPM (Figure 3.24).

Figure 3.23. Inpatient Costs in Cincinnati Relative to Reference Markets

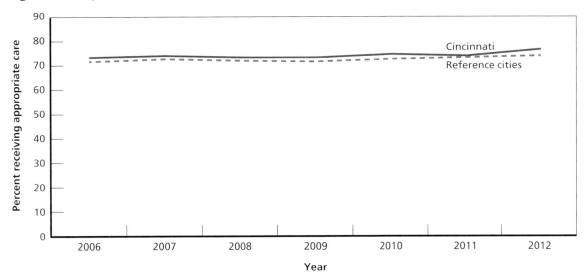

SOURCE: Authors' analysis of MarketScan data, 2006–2012.
RAND *RR729-3.23*

Figure 3.24. Total PMPM Costs in Cincinnati Relative to Reference Markets

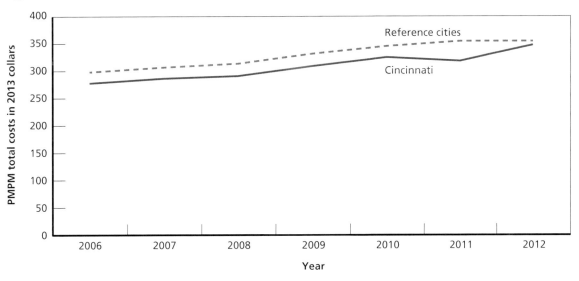

SOURCE: Authors' analysis of MarketScan data, 2006–2012.
RAND *RR729-3.24*

Results

Sensitivity Analysis

As pointed out earlier, we conducted separate analyses for residents that were always in an HDHP and for those who were never in such plans. Our assumption is that the residents who did not change coverage type—and, therefore, did not experience a change in incentives to seek care—would give us a better representation of the true intervention effect. Overall, those sensitivity analyses yielded similar results to our main analyses, except that among the population always enrolled in an HDHP, the intervention was associated with different patterns in outpatient and prescription utilizations (see shaded cells in Table 3.1). We present the detailed results of the sensitivity analyses for outpatient utilization and costs and prescription drug utilization and costs in both populations.

Table 3.1. Sensitivity Analysis: Intervention Effects on Quality of Care, Health Care Utilization, and Health Care Cost

Domain	Outcome Metrics	Always in an HDHP			Never in an HDHP		
		2010	2011	2012	2010	2011	2012
Access to primary care	Adults' access to preventive/ambulatory health services	—	—	—	—	—	↓
	Children's and adolescents' access to primary care practitioners	—	—	↓	—	—	↓
Chronic care	Percentage of patients using ARBs/ACE inhibitors who receive appropriate monitoring	—	—	—	—	↓	—
	Percentage of patients on diuretics receiving appropriate monitoring	—	—	—	—	↓	—
	Percentage of asthma patients receiving appropriate medications	↓	—	—	—	—	—
	Percentage of diabetic patients receiving HbA1c testing	—	—	—	—	—	—
	Percentage of diabetic patients receiving LDL-c testing	—	—	—	—	—	—
	Percentage of patients with low back pain who did not have an imaging within 28 days of the diagnosis	—	—	—	—	—	—
Preventable admissions and ED visits	Ambulatory care sensitive inpatient admissions	↓	—	—	—	—	↓
	Inpatient readmissions within 30 days of discharge	—	—	—	—	—	—
	Potentially avoidable ED visits	—	—	—	—	—	↓
Outpatient	Office-based primary care visits	—	↑	—	—	—	↓
	Outpatient PMPM cost	—	—	—	—	↓	—
Prescription drug	Prescription drug fills	↑	—	—	↓	↓	↓
	Prescription drug PMPM cost	—	↓	—	—	↓	↓
Emergency care	ED visits	—	—	—	—	↑	—
	ED PMPM cost	—	—	—	—	—	—
Inpatient care	Inpatient admissions	—	—	—	—	—	—
	Inpatient PMPM cost	—	—	—	—	—	—
Total cost	Total PMPM Cost	—	—	—	—	—	—

NOTE: The table shows the changes in Cincinnati relative to the reference cities. — indicates no statistically significant findings. ↑ represents a statistically significant increase in Cincinnati relative to the reference cities (p≤0.05). Compared to the reference cities, an outcome metric may increase more or decline less in Cincinnati. ↓ represents a statistically significant decrease in Cincinnati relative to the reference cities (p≤0.05). The shaded cells show the results that are different from the main analysis. Compared to the reference cities, an outcome metric may increase less or decline more in Cincinnati.

Results

In contrast to the results in the overall population, the Cincinnati residents who were always in an HDHP showed a significant increase in outpatient services and prescription utilization, but a significant decrease in prescription costs relative to the reference cities.

Residents who were always in an HDHP reduced their utilization of outpatient services over the course of the study, but this decline was significantly less for Cincinnati residents in 2011 relative to the reference cities. As shown in Figure 3.25, outpatient utilization decreased over the course of the intervention in the HDHP population, going from an average of 1,744 visits per 1,000 member years in the baseline period to 1,505 visits per 1,000 member years in 2012. The differential between Cincinnati and the reference cities increased significantly, from an average of 17.5 more visits per 1,000 member years in Cincinnati than the reference cities in the baseline period to 53 more visits per 1,000 member years in Cincinnati in 2011. While utilization was decreasing, outpatient costs in this population were increasing in both Cincinnati and the reference cities; however, there was no significant change in the difference between costs in Cincinnati and the reference cities (Figure 3.26).

The prescription drug utilization for the population always in an HDHP in Cincinnati had a small increase over the course of the intervention and roughly constant costs, aside from a slight reduction in 2011. During the baseline period, residents in Cincinnati had 5,014 prescriptions per 1,000 member years, which in 2012 rose to 5,479 prescriptions per 1,000 member years. Cincinnati residents had higher prescription drug utilization than the reference markets throughout the study period, with an average of 635 more prescriptions per 1,000 member years in the baseline period. During the intervention years, the difference between Cincinnati and the reference cities was significantly above the baseline average in 2010, with 883 more prescriptions in Cincinnati per 1,000 member years than the reference cities (Figure 3.27).

Figure 3.25. Outpatient Utilization for the Population Always Enrolled in an HDHP in Cincinnati Relative to Reference Markets

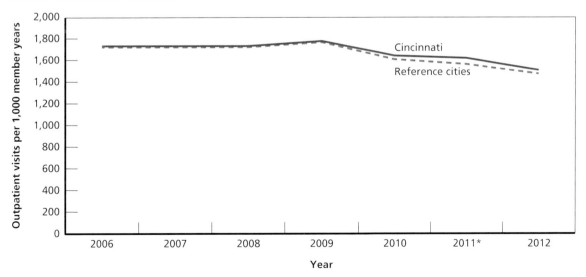

SOURCE: Authors' analysis of MarketScan data, 2006–2012.
NOTE: *p≤0.05 for the intervention effect.
RAND *RR729-3.25*

Results

Figure 3.26. Outpatient Costs for the Population Always Enrolled in an HDHP in Cincinnati Relative to Reference Markets

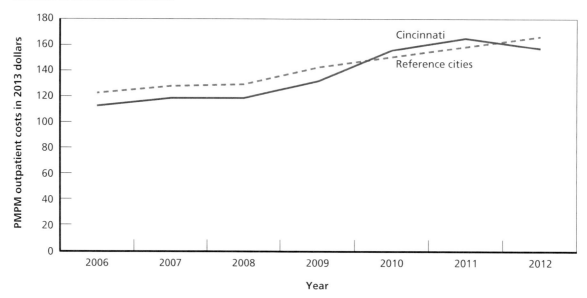

SOURCE: Authors' analysis of MarketScan data, 2006–2012.
RAND RR729-3.26

Figure 3.27. Prescription Drug Utilization for the Population Always Enrolled in an HDHP in Cincinnati Relative to Reference Markets

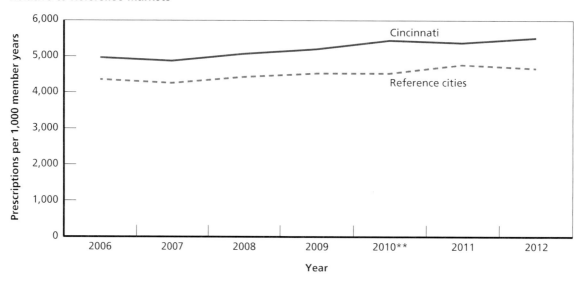

SOURCE: Authors' analysis of MarketScan data, 2006–2012.
NOTE: **p≤0.01 for the intervention effect.
RAND RR729-3.27

Prescription drug costs in Cincinnati were, on average, $9.06 PMPM higher than in the reference cities in the baseline period. That difference shrank in each intervention year, and the change was significant in 2011 when the difference dropped to an estimated $0.63 less PMPM in Cincinnati than in the reference cities (Figure 3.28).

Figure 3.28. Prescription Drug Costs for the Population Always Enrolled in an HDHP in Cincinnati Relative to Reference Markets

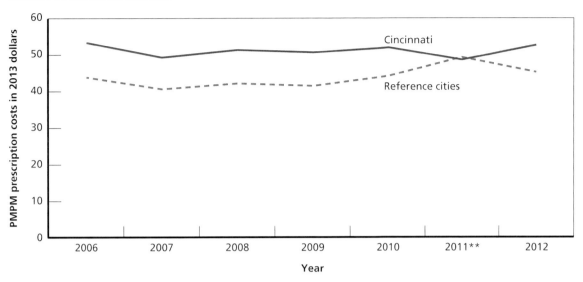

SOURCE: Authors' analysis of SMART BRFSS data, 2006–2012.
NOTES: **p≤0.01 for the intervention effect.
RAND *RR729-3.28*

Consistent with increased prescription utilization and decreased prescription costs, the cost per prescription also decreased over time in Cincinnati relative to the reference cities. Compared with a slight increase from $115.2 in the preintervention years to $119.3 in the intervention years in the reference cities, the cost per prescription in Cincinnati declined from $122.3 to $113.0.

NEVER IN AN HDHP

Outpatient utilization and costs for residents who were never enrolled in an HDHP followed trends similar to the Cincinnati population as a whole. In this subgroup, the number of outpatient visits decreased in each year of the intervention, from an average of 1,685 visits per 1,000 member years at baseline to 1,505 visits per 1,000 member years in 2012 (Figure 3.29). Cincinnati residents had between 21 and 25 more visits per 1,000 member years than the reference cities in each year of the study except 2012, when Cincinnati residents had an estimated 111 fewer outpatient visits per 1,000 member years than the reference cities. This was a significant change from the baseline difference. Costs in Cincinnati and the reference cities trended upward over the course of the study. There was a significant change in 2011, when Cincinnati's PMPM costs were $23.53 less PMPM than the reference cities, compared with an average baseline differential of $6.03 less PMPM in Cincinnati (Figure 3.30).

Prescription drug utilization and costs in the population never enrolled in an HDHP followed a very similar trend to the main results. In the baseline period, Cincinnati averaged 28 prescriptions more than the reference cities per 1,000 member years, but the difference changed significantly relative to the difference at baseline, to 57 fewer prescriptions in Cincinnati per 1,000

Results

31

Figure 3.29. Outpatient Utilization for the Population Never Enrolled in an HDHP in Cincinnati Relative to Reference Markets

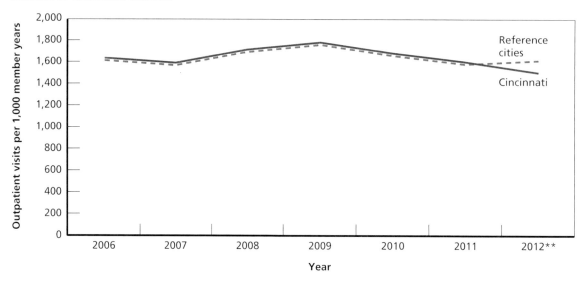

SOURCE: Authors' analysis of MarketScan data, 2006–2012.
NOTE: **p≤0.01 for the intervention effect.
RAND RR729-3.29

Figure 3.30. Outpatient Costs for the Population Never Enrolled in an HDHP in Cincinnati Relative to Reference Markets

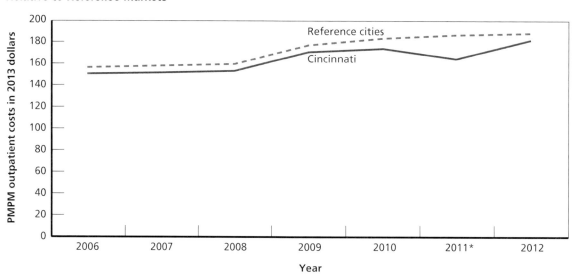

SOURCE: Authors' analysis of MarketScan data, 2006–2012.
NOTE: *p≤0.05 for the intervention effect.
RAND RR729-3.30

member years in 2010, 783 fewer prescriptions in Cincinnati per 1,000 member years in 2011, and 875 fewer prescriptions in Cincinnati per 1,000 member years in 2012 (Figure 3.31). The decreases in prescription drug utilization translated into significant differential differences in costs in 2011

Figure 3.31. Prescription Drug Utilization for the Population Never Enrolled in an HDHP in Cincinnati Relative to Reference Markets

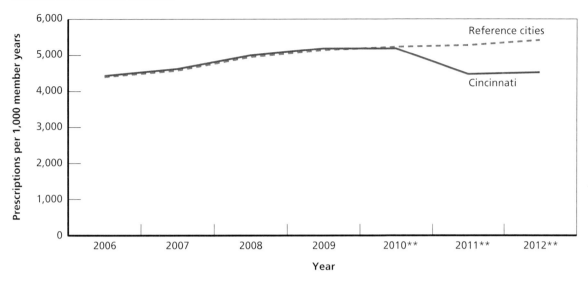

SOURCE: Authors' analysis of MarketScan data, 2006–2012.
NOTE: **p≤0.01 for the intervention effect.
RAND *RR729-3.31*

Figure 3.32. Prescription Drug Costs for the Population Never Enrolled in an HDHP in Cincinnati Relative to Reference Markets

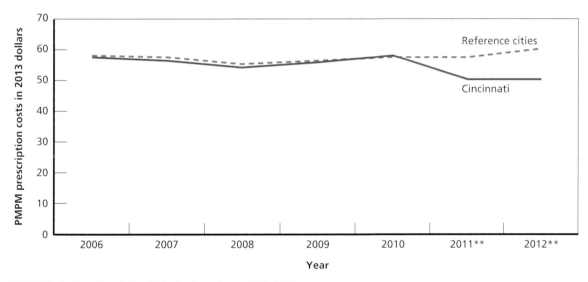

SOURCE: Authors' analysis of MarketScan data, 2006–2012.
NOTE: **p≤0.01 for the intervention effect.
RAND *RR729-3.32*

and 2012 relative to the baseline difference between Cincinnati and the reference cities (Figure 3.32).

Results

4

Discussion

Summary of Findings

The Healthy Communities Initiative in Cincinnati combines primary care innovation, care coordination, the introduction of a health information exchange, public reporting of provider performance data, payment innovation, and targeted initiatives to improve care for patients with asthma and diabetes. We report on the early results of this ambitious initiative three years into the intervention. The analysis is based on a comparison of market-level trends for health status, health care quality, and cost and utilization of care in Cincinnati relative to 15 comparable reference markets. In addition, we used statistical techniques to account for market-level and resident-level differences between those markets to isolate the intervention effect. The findings are summarized in Table 4.1.

BETTER HEALTH

The Healthy Communities Initiative in Cincinnati was associated with improved employee productivity as indicated by a decrease in work hours missed due to illness, which translates into about 140,000 working hours or about 70 FTE employees in 2012. Nonetheless, the intervention was not linked to significant improvements in residents' health and health behaviors.

BETTER CARE

We find improvements in preventable hospital admissions and readmissions that point to better care coordination, particularly for higher-risk patients. At the same time, use of primary and outpatient care, prescription drugs, and adherence to evidence-based recommendations for chronic care management all decreased in Cincinnati compared to the reference cities. Use of ED services increased.

LOWER COST

These changes in utilization patterns did not translate into significant changes in overall health care costs, while spending on prescription drugs declined.

Discussion

Table 4.1. Main Analysis: Intervention Effects on Health, Quality of Care, Health Care Utilization, and Health Care Cost

Domain	Outcome Metrics	Intervention Years		
		2010	2011	2012
Health	Self-reported health status	—	—	—
	Obesity	—	—	—
	Smoking	—	—	—
	Binge drinking	—	—	—
Productivity	Any missed work due to illness	—	—	↓
	Work hours missed due to illness	—	—	↓
Access to primary care	Adults' access to preventive/ambulatory health services	—	—	↓
	Children's and adolescents' access to primary care practitioners	↓	↓	↓
Chronic care	Percentage of patients using ARBs/ACE inhibitors who receive appropriate monitoring	—	↓	↓
	Percentage of patients on diuretics receiving appropriate monitoring	—	↓	↓
	Percentage of asthma patients receiving appropriate medications	↓	↓	—
	Percentage of diabetic patients receiving HbA1c testing	—	↓	—
	Percentage of diabetic patients receiving LDL-c testing	—	—	—
	Percentage of patients with low back pain without imaging within 28 days of the diagnosis	—	—	—
Preventable admissions and ED visits	Ambulatory care sensitive inpatient admissions	—	—	↓
	Inpatient readmissions within 30 days of discharge	↓	—	—
	Potentially avoidable ED visits	—	—	—
Outpatient	Office-based primary care visits	↓	↓	↓
	Outpatient PMPM cost	—	—	—
Prescription drug	Prescription drug fills	↓	↓	↓
	Prescription drug PMPM cost	—	↓	↓
Emergency care	ED visits	↓	↓	↓
	ED PMPM cost	—	↓	—
Inpatient care	Inpatient admissions	—	—	—
	Inpatient PMPM cost	—	—	—
Total cost	Total PMPM Cost	—	—	—

NOTE: The table shows the changes in Cincinnati relative to the reference cities. — indicates no statistically significant findings.
↑ represents a statistically significant increase in Cincinnati relative to the reference cities (p≤0.05). Compared to the reference cities, an outcome metric may increase more or decline less in Cincinnati. ↓ represents a statistically significant decrease in Cincinnati relative to the reference cities (p≤0.05). Compared to the reference cities, an outcome metric may increase less or decline more in Cincinnati.

Discussion

BETTER HEALTH

The absence of a strong effect of the intervention on health status indicators, such as body weight and smoking rates, is not surprising. First, it may take a period of longer than three years to observe significant changes in health behaviors and health status. In addition, the intervention did not explicitly target health-related behaviors; rather, it largely focused on improving medical care. Even well-resourced and personalized interventions, such as workplace wellness programs, are known to have only a limited effect on health-related behaviors, such as smoking cessation and physical activities (Mattke et al., 2013a). It is thus to be expected that improvements in health are unlikely to materialize as a "side effect" of the interventions. However, we did find a differential decrease in illness-related work loss in Cincinnati. While instances of sick leave declined in both Cincinnati and the 15 reference markets after 2009, presumably as a consequence of the recession, the trend was much stronger in Cincinnati and reached statistical difference in 2012, the third year of the intervention. As the trend is adjusted for differences in age structure and burden of disease between Cincinnati and the reference markets, we interpret it as an early sign of improved health of the workforce.

BETTER CARE

We find that the Healthy Communities Initiative in Cincinnati was significantly associated with reductions in hospital readmissions and ambulatory care sensitive hospital admissions, suggesting improved care coordination and better post-discharge management for higher-risk patients. During the intervention period, the Greater Cincinnati Health Council's Accountable Care Transformation group engaged 21 hospitals in reducing readmissions and improving care coordination after a hospital admission, which could contribute to the decline in hospital readmissions. Additionally, the 2012 introduction of the HealthBridge alert system is likely to have contributed to this result, as it notifies primary care providers if one of their patients has been admitted to a hospital or visited an ED, thus facilitating planning and management of care transitions. As mentioned, 87 sites were running and 26,000 alerts had been sent by October 2012 (U.S. Department of Health and Human Services and Office of the National Coordinator for Health Information Technology, November 2012).

At the same time, the observed decline in use of primary and outpatient care and prescription drugs is counterintuitive, as is the lower adherence to evidence-based recommendations for chronic care management and increased ED use. If the intervention worked as expected, we would observe increased use of primary care and prescriptions, improved chronic disease management, and fewer inpatient admissions and ED visits.

It should be emphasized that a *finding of no effect* would not have been entirely surprising, as the intervention is still in its early stages. While formally in its third year at the time of the evaluation, many of the more fundamental changes are just beginning to take effect. Better access to high-quality primary care through the promulgation of the PCMH concept is one of the cornerstones of the initiative. As of mid-2013, 84 practices in the Cincinnati MSA have obtained NCQA Level 3 PCMH recognition, representing about 24 percent of the primary care providers in Cincinnati. Practices that have only recently obtained their PCMH designation may not have reached their full potential. A recent study of a medical home pilot in Pennsylvania detected no significant effects on utilization or cost of care, and only a limited effect on quality of care, over a three-year intervention (Friedberg et al., 2014). Similarly, a new alert system of the HealthBridge health information exchange was implemented in 2012.

Finding *opposite trends* from what we expected is surprising, though it can likely be explained by the wide adoption of HDHPs in Cincinnati relative to the reference markets during these first three years of the Healthy Communities Initiative. The share of HDHPs in Cincinnati more than doubled, from 13.4 percent in 2009 to 28.5 percent in 2012, but only increased from 7.5 percent to 10.8 percent in the reference cities during the same time frame. As HDHPs shift responsibility for health care costs to plan members, they have profound impacts on utilization patterns. Prior literature suggests that HDHPs reduce health care spending by 5–14 percent on average, although the effect varies across employers (Bundorf, 2012). Cost savings from HDHPs are primarily due to reductions in prescription cost and outpatient cost. HDHPs have no consistent effect on inpatient admissions, and they have modest to no reductions in preventive services use when they are exempted from the deductible and significant reductions when they are not. Consumers in HDHPs may indiscriminately reduce utilization. One study focusing on the adoption of HDHPs and consumer-directed health plans found that both spending and preventive care utilization went down in the first year, even though preventive care did not count against the deductible (Buntin et al., 2011). To explain their findings, Buntin et al. suggested that the high deductible may generally deter patients from seeking care or that patients may not have fully understood the exemption of preventive care from their deductible in the first year after adoption of an HDHP. If the latter is the case, the population in an HDHP may increase its utilization of preventive services as they begin to understand their benefit design better. Another study found significant reductions in outpatient visits and general laboratory tests, but not preventive laboratory tests, for people who switch to an HDHP (Reddy et al., 2014). The reduction in outpatient visits reflected decreases in visits for both higher- and lower-priority chronic conditions. There is also evidence that people in HDHPs are less likely to visit an ED, to be hospitalized (Wharam et al., 2007), and to use prescription drugs (Greene et al., 2008). The impacts of HDHPs may be particularly pronounced on sicker patients, because they require more care, and on patients with lower socioeconomic status (Committee on Child Health Financing, 2014).

To account for the adoption of HDHPs in our analysis, we included an indicator for HDHP in all the models and also conducted sensitivity analyses using the individuals who were always in an HDHP or never in an HDHP during 2006–2012 under the assumption that these individuals did not experience a significant change in cost-sharing arrangements and thus would not likely change their care seeking behavior. The results in those subsamples were, however, largely similar to those in the overall population. One possible explanation is that the rapid adoption of HDHPs in the Cincinnati market affected not only the individuals in an HDHP but also those not in an HDHP. This hypothesis is consistent with prior research showing that providers tend to orient their practice patterns to the average or modal insurance coverage in their catchment areas (Glied and Zivin, 2002; Hu and Reuben, 2002; Landon, 2004). A caveat, however, is that this body of literature is primarily based on experience in managed care, which typically imposes financial incentives on providers, whereas in this case, HDHPs primarily influence patients' care-seeking behaviors. It is also possible that other unobserved factors, such as new provider payment arrangements, led to the similar findings in individuals never enrolled in an HDHP to those in the full sample.

LOWER COST

Those changes in use of care did not translate into changes in overall cost of care during the first three years of the intervention. This finding can be explained by the fact that payment innovations—which, based on prior research, are the most likely instrument to reduce overall cost—were implemented only recently in Cincinnati. In the Cincinnati-Dayton region, 75 practices have joined the Centers for Medicaid and Medicare Services' CPC Initiative, in which payers offer bonus payments to primary care providers who effectively coordinate patient care. In addition, Cincinnati's Mercy Health System is involved in a national payment reform pilot with the CMS, the Medicare Shared Savings Program, but the initiative became operational only in the fall of 2012.

Limitations

There are several limitations to this analysis. First and foremost, unobservable differences between Cincinnati and the 15 reference markets, as well as their respective residents, may have influenced our results. The CPS and BRFSS data did not allow us to track individuals over time, which might have reduced our ability to detect the intervention effect. In addition, we were not able to control for the changes in the health care delivery system of other markets during the study period. This could have led to an underestimation of the effect of the interventions implemented in Cincinnati. Further, no data were available on nontraditional forms of care delivery in PCMHs, such as phone consultations or electronic exchanges between providers and patients. It is likely that nontraditional services substitute for in-person physician visits. If this is true, office-based primary care visits are not a good measure for quality improvement within the PCMH environment because a decrease in office-based primary care visits may not be interpreted as a decline in access to primary care. Moreover, we were not able to tease out the potential selection in HDHP participation. GE, as one of the largest employers in Cincinnati, required all salaried employees to join an HDHP in 2010 and required all production employees to do the same in 2012. But we are not sure whether an HDHP plan was the only option offered by other employers in Cincinnati or employers in the reference cities. This potential selection bias may have confounded our sensitivity analyses for those always or never enrolled in an HDHP plan.

Discussion

Conclusions

WE CONDUCTED THE FIRST QUANTITATIVE EVALUATION ON THE HEALTHY COMMUNITIES INITIATIVE in Cincinnati for its first three intervention years. Overall, our findings were largely inconclusive because of the concomitant marketwide shift to HDHPs and the early stage of the intervention.

Transitioning to HDHPs is known to have profound effects on care-seeking behaviors—particularly immediately after a change in benefit design, as plan members adapt to the new incentives. As the share of HDHP plans more than doubled in Cincinnati during our analysis period, it may have concealed intervention effects. As the level of HDHP penetration in Cincinnati stabilizes—and, thus, the effect of switching to HDHPs on utilizations and costs decreases—analyzing additional years of data will allow us to disentangle the effects of the intervention from the effects of benefit design changes.

As key components of the intervention (such as payment redesign, PCMHs, and the HealthBridge alert notification) were still being fully implemented during the period of analysis, the intervention will not have been able to take full effect. We did find some encouraging signs that better care coordination bears fruit, such as less illness-related work loss and fewer avoidable hospital admissions and readmissions. These early impacts suggest that the initiative may succeed in improving care, lowering cost, and improving health status if given sufficient time. Therefore, a future evaluation of the Healthy Communities Initiative in Cincinnati will be able to assess a more mature program, leverage more data, and result in more conclusive findings.

Conclusions

Bibliography

AHRQ Quality Indicators (2001). *Guide to prevention quality indicators: Hospital admission for ambulatory care sensitive conditions.* Department of Health and Human Services Agency for Healthcare Research and Quality.

Bundorf, M. K. (2012). Consumer-directed health plans: Do they deliver? *POLICY 1*:6.

Buntin, M., Haviland, A. M., McDevitt, R., and Sood, N. (2011). Healthcare spending and preventive care in high-deductible and consumer-directed health plans. *American Journal of Managed Care, 17*(3), 222–230.

CDC—*See* Centers for Disease Control and Prevention.

Centers for Disease Control and Prevention (2012). *Behavioral risk factor surveillance system survey data.* Atlanta: U.S. Department of Health and Human Services.

Charlson, M. E., Pompei, P., Ales, K. L., and MacKenzie C. R. (1987). A new method of classifying prognostic comorbidity in longitudinal studies: development and validation. *Journal of Chronic Diseases 40*(5), 373–383.

Committee on Child Health Financing (2014). High-Deductible Health Plans. *Pediatrics 133*(5), e1461–e1470. As of August 6, 2014: http://pediatrics.aappublications.org/content/133/5/e1461.abstract

Deyo, R. A., Cherkin, D. C., and Ciol, M. A. (1992). Adapting a clinical comorbidity index for use with ICD-9-CM administrative databases. *Journal of Clinical Epidemiology 45*(6), 613–619.

Friedberg, M. W., Schneider, E. C., Rosenthal, M. B., Volpp, K. G., and Werner, R. M. (2014). Association between participation in a multipayer medical home intervention and changes in quality, utilization, and costs of care. *JAMA 311*(8), 815–825.

Glied, S., and Zivin, J. G. (2002). How do doctors behave when some (but not all) of their patients are in managed care? *Journal of Health Economics 21*(2), 337–353.

Greene, J., Hibbard, J., Murray, J. F., Teutsch, S. M., and Berger, M. L. (2008). The impact of consumer-directed health plans on prescription drug use. *Health Affairs 27*(4), 1111–1119. As of August 6, 2014: http://content.healthaffairs.org/content/27/4/1111.abstract

Hibbard, J. H., Stockard, J., and Tusler, M. (2005). Hospital performance reports: Impact on quality, market share, and reputation. *Health Affairs 24*(4), 1150–1160.

Hu, P., and Reuben, D. B. (2002). Effects of managed care on the length of time that elderly patients spend with physicians during ambulatory visits: National Ambulatory Medical Care Survey. *Medical Care 40*(7), 606–613.

IHI—*See* Institute for Healthcare Improvement.

Institute for Healthcare Improvement (2013). *IHI Triple Aim initiative.*

Jackson, G. L., Powers, B. J., Chatterjee, R., Bettger, J. P., Kemper, A. R., Hasselblad, V., et al. (2013). The Patient-Centered Medical Home: A systematic review. *Annals of Internal Medicine 158*(3), 169–178. As of August 6, 2014: http://dx.doi.org/10.7326/0003-4819-158-3-201302050-00579

Landon, B. E. (2004). Commentary on "Penetrating the 'Black Box': Financial incentives for enhancing the quality of physician services," by Douglas A. Conrad and Jon B. Christianson. *Medical Care Research and Review 61*(3 suppl), 69S–75S.

Lee, B. K., Lessler, J., and Stuart, E. A. (2011). Weight trimming and propensity score weighting. *PloS one 6*(3), e18174.

Mattke, S., Liu, H., Caloyeras, J., Huang, C. Y., Van Busum, K. R., Khodyakov, D., et al. (2013). *Workplace wellness programs study.* Santa Monica, Calif.: RAND Corporation, RR-254-DOL. As of August 6, 2014: http://www.rand.org/pubs/research_reports/RR254.html

Mattke, S., Sorbero, M., et al. (2013). *An impact study of the local health collaborative in Cincinnati.* Santa Monica, Calif.: RAND Corporation. Not available to the general public.

NCQA—*See* National Committee for Quality Assurance.

National Committee for Quality Assurance (2011). *HEDIS 2011 technical specifications (Vol. 2).*

Oehlert, G. W. (1992). A note on the delta method. *The American Statistician 46*(1), 27–29.

Radley, D. C., and Commonwealth Fund (2012). *Rising to the challenge: Results from a scorecard on local health system performance, 2012.* Commonwealth Fund.

Reddy, S. R., Ross-Degnan, D., Zaslavsky, A. M., Soumerai, S. B., and Wharam, J. F. (2014). Impact of a high-deductible health plan on outpatient visits and associated diagnostic tests. *Medical Care 52*(1), 86–92.

Rosenthal, T. C. (2008). The medical home: Growing evidence to support a new approach to primary care. *J Am Board Fam Med 21*(5), 427–440. As of August 6, 2014: http://www.ncbi.nlm.nih.gov/pubmed/18772297

Stürmer, T., Rothman, K. J., Avorn, J., and Glynn, R. J. (2010). Treatment effects in the presence of unmeasured confounding: Dealing with observations in the tails of the propensity score distribution—a simulation study. *American Journal of Epidemiology.*

Truven Health Analytics (2012). *MarketScan® research databases.* Ann Arbor, Mich.

U.S. Department of Health and Human Services and Office of the National Coordinator for Health Information Technology (November 2012) *Fact Sheet: Greater Cincinnati Beacon Collaboration.*

U.S. Census Bureau and the Bureau of Labor Statistics (2012). *Current populations survey.*

Wharam, J. F., Landon, B. E., Galbraith, A. A., Kleinman, K. P., Soumerai, S. B., and Ross-Degnan, D. (2007). Emergency department use and subsequent hospitalizations among members of a high-deductible health plan. *JAMA 297*(10), 1093–1102.

Bibliography